PRAISE FOR GORDON BOSWORTH'S WHY DOES IT HURT?

'I've been seeing Gordon since April 2023, and he quickly became an integral part of my performance set-up. His unrivalled ability to solve the problems my body presents as an elite sub 10 second 100m sprinter is invaluable. Regular visits to his clinic have become a staple in my programme to ensure my body remains mechanically sound and able to express itself without hindrance. I'm grateful for his continued support and would recommend him to all who desire to first understand the body and how best to optimise it for performance.'

– Eugene Amo-Dadzie,
GB 100m sprinter

'Having worked in football for almost 40 years, I have never met anyone more knowledgeable and capable of solving the unsolvable. His personality and willingness to understand the rules that govern football dressing rooms allowed him to be accepted as one of the group, not an easy challenge! I completely trust Gordon (aka the Guru) in his clinical diagnoses and more importantly, as a friend.'

–Eric Black, Ex-professional footballer,
Coach and Manager

Why Does it Hurt?

The Musculoskeletal Insidious Onset Conundrum

Why Does it Hurt?

The Musculoskeletal Insidious Onset Conundrum

GORDON BOSWORTH

CONTENTS

INTRODUCTION   7

1. WHAT IS HEALTH?   9

2. INSIDIOUS ONSET PAIN   17

3. A MEETING TO REMEMBER   27

4. RELATIONSHIPS   41

5. PUBLIC AND PRIVATE   63

6. THE EMERGENT BODY   69

7. AN INTEGRATED APPROACH   83

8. THE NEXT GENERATION   97

CONCLUSIONS   105

INTRODUCTION

I'm sure I am not alone in reflecting back on my life and the time I've spent building a body of work and wondering how and if it might be remembered.

These reflections prompted me to start writing some of my thoughts down and sharing a bit about my life to date as a way of helping me understand how I've gotten to where I am today. If my observations can also help or shape future generations, then so much the better. At the very least, this book can stand as a testament to my contribution to society.

Why Does It Hurt? is intended as a foundational and philosophical text, but my goal is to write additional books with a more technical bias that focus specifically on the application of this philosophy. In order to understand how I have arrived at this point in my life, it was important to give you, the reader, some background.

We all develop our own philosophies over the course of our lives. This is mine. I hope you find it interesting.

Why Does it Hurt? Is dedicated to my wife and family, who have stood by my side throughout.

1. WHAT IS HEALTH?

The body hates inefficiency: it's something we have in common. When something's not working, it will communicate, overcompensate, or stop working altogether until the problem's solved. There is much that we can ignore or put off doing in our lives – the dripping bathroom tap we really ought to get fixed, the strange noise coming from the car, the email reminders to renew a gym membership – but what we cannot ignore is pain. There is no more effective way for the body to tell us it's not happy than pain. For most of us, it's a daily occurrence in some form or another: the stubbed toe, the creaking hip, the headache. These can be mild or severe, but it's the latter camp where I've chosen to pitch my tent.

MSK therapy is like detective work: we follow the evidence. Even when the body is inefficient, it can still function effectively for a period of time. Sometimes, that smoking gun is staring us in the face, and we catch – or treat – the culprit red-handed. Sometimes, things are a little more complicated, and we're faced with irrelevancies, red herrings and circumstantial evidence. But we always aim to build the picture piece by piece, most notably through conversation. For me, listening to a patient is as important as examining them. It doesn't matter if they downplay the problem or scale it up: every person who walks through my door is there for a reason, and those reasons differ. The relationships we form in the first 10 minutes are often as important as anything else in forming a diagnosis. Without realising it, my team and I become very quickly versed in the intricacies of human psychology, first and foremost. It's about trust. It's multidisciplinary, this line of work – and that, besides so much else, is why I love what I do.

This book is for patients and practitioners alike: it's also for anyone interested in furthering their understanding of how their body responds to and manages injuries. My aim here is to bring 40 years of experience to bear in educating not only the next generation of people like me but also the people they treat. We live in a fast-paced, hyper-accelerated society, a culture of movement and frenetic energy. Our recent brushes with lockdown may have curbed this in some, but for the majority of us, life continues at the same breakneck speed, with often little regard for our general health until the damage is well and truly done. We have no patience. When an Amazon delivery driver can be at the door mere hours after we click 'confirm', there is little room in our collective psyche now for three-month waiting lists, for resting and waiting for the body to work its magic, for time to simply pass. More so than ever before, I think, our expectations far outweigh our bodies' capabilities or the speed at which they were designed to move. It can be easy to forget that we're not robots – not yet anyway – and our programming has been inbuilt, finessed, fine-tuned and adapted over millennia. It's not something that can be rushed, however much we'd like to rush it.

This is not just a book about me, and yet it's important to lay out why I am where I am and how I came to be here. Following a successful 16-year stint at the Royal Air Force's

Physical Education Branch, during which I trained at Queen Elizabeth's Military Hospital in Woolwich, I moved to the RAF School of Physiotherapy and qualified in 1983. Since then, my work has taken me far and wide, from tours of duty on various units to head of rehabilitation at the Police Rehab Centre at Goring-on-Thames.

Since moving into private practice, I've served as medical lead and chief physiotherapist for various Olympic teams and as a consultant to several professional football and rugby teams. I founded the Bosworth Clinic 10 years ago in a bid to change the way injuries were managed and patients advised to manage their symptoms and to provide courses to those hoping to enter our field. We see hundreds of patients every month, presenting with a whole plethora of different complaints, and it is this diversity and experience I would like to document.

I want to see us changing the way we gather information from the outset and stop regarding the body as an exact science. It's much more like an art form: malleable, ever-changing and given to all sorts of caprice.

I do not profess to have all the answers – not by any means. But I have some, and my training continues to enable greater knowledge and appreciation for the many messages our bodies attempt to give us every day. We can do better, both in public and in private practice, and thus transform the quality of life for millions. Less than a hundred years ago, patients frequently died of ailments we now regard as eminently curable: infections, polio, whooping cough, tuberculosis, measles and scarlet fever. The creation of the NHS in 1948 and the introduction of antibiotics to our medical arsenal changed a great deal when it came to citizens' chances of survival. Now, treatment was no longer dependent on the depth of one's pockets or on a strict regime of bloodletting, herbs and potions. We had combat weapons. But what of the muscular-skeletal system? Of course, we have seen huge advances here, too, but not – perhaps – to the same degree as in acute medicine. And this is to be expected: a blood infection remains potentially fatal if untreated, while a broken leg or fractured pelvis is usually not.

And so I return to our all-too-prevalent habits of putting our problems off, of waiting and hoping for some relief. It doesn't need to be like this, and MSK therapy provides so much of the solution. So let me take you through it, step by step, and I hope that in doing so, this book will prove instructional and helpful.

This isn't a book about me, but in describing the experience of working, in the main, with athletes and various professional sporting teams, I will inevitably reference my own findings and reflections. On moving into private practice, I began to move away from my prior work with military personnel and police rehabilitation.

I spent three years as head of rehabilitation at the Goring-on-Thames centre, and honestly, if I'd taken the job now, it's likely I would have stayed forever. It was a fascinating place to cut one's teeth, to really get into the heart of what the job entailed and to work with a wide variety of clients with different issues. Sports injuries are one thing – and these are most commonly what I focus on nowadays – but the problems associated with the military and the police are a different ball game. Now, I was working with clients who'd experienced direct trauma from attacks – they'd been injured in the line of duty – and who needed to be made fit again to retain the jobs they so loved.

It is terrible to imagine the pain of being shot or stabbed, but perhaps even more difficult is the post-operative recovery, the inevitable trauma therapy that is required and the hours of attempting to navigate what has happened to you. In the police force, physios will deal with stabbings, gunshot wounds and most commonly contact injuries. With knife crime on the rise across the UK, it is depressingly common for not only the victims and perpetrators of such attacks to become seriously hurt but those who protect them, too.

In the military, it is also common to see MSK therapy requirements delivered on the front line and, more commonly, once troops return from active duty: these are often the gravest, most intensely debilitating injuries, such as traumatic amputations. The prevalence of IEDs, for instance, in recent wars abroad, has seen a marked increase in soldiers needing extensive and ongoing MSK therapy. There are also injuries associated with ejection seats in Jets and, of course, the terrible effect of burns.

I enjoyed the challenges this work presented enormously, but it's so important to think through your career options carefully to prevent yourself from becoming stale to ensure that each new opportunity represents one for growth. I enjoyed the work immensely but found, after a time, that I was de-skilling: I was in my early 30s, and I wasn't able to really spread my wings. At the Police Convalescent Centre in Goring, Most of the reason for this revolved around the first 10 days after an injury: we just didn't see patients beyond that point. As a result, it was almost impossible to plan in the middle- or long-term. Everything was early assessments, and though my skills in that department came on in leaps and bounds, I just felt I wasn't getting the experience I needed across the board.

It was around this time that I began to become involved with athletes and sports teams more widely. Between 1996 and 2006, including four years as performance director, I served as the senior governing body physiotherapist to the British bobsleigh and bob-skeleton team.

Subsequently, I worked as a member of the Great Britain teams at the Winter Olympic Games in Nagano, Japan, in 1998, Salt Lake City in 2002, and Italy's Torino in 2006. I've been the medical lead for the Canadian speed skating team at the Vancouver Olympic Games (2010) and chief physiotherapist to UK Athletics / British Athletics at the London Olympic Games in 2012. I attended the Olympic holding camp with Canada in Sochi, Russia (2014) and the Pyeongchang Winter Games in Korea (2018), again with Canada and recently Tokyo 2020 with Great Britain as part of the Athletics Medical team.

Football is, as we know, our national sport: I've been lucky enough to work as a consultant with teams from Wigan to Liverpool, Bolton, Derby County, Queen's Park Rangers and Sunderland. More recently, Brentford and Rangers. Although I'm sure many young people would relish the opportunity to work as football physios specifically, unfortunately, no such job exists. All physios need to be able to work across a broad range of sports and disciplines. However, football presents such fascinating challenges.

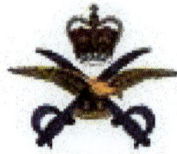

The RAF PTI Badge. I graduated RAF St Athan School of Physical Training in 1977. My first very proud moment.

2. INSIDIOUS ONSET PAIN

While acute pain – the sort that makes people book doctors' appointments or head to A&E – grabs our immediate attention, many other kinds do not. We might notice aches and niggles in a roundabout, generalised sort of way and dismiss them as par for the course, blame a recent game of tennis or put them down to ageing. Over time, these ever-so-slightly problematic issues become steadily more and more painful. We find we can't climb the stairs as easily, pick up our suitcase, go for a run.

One of the main issues with any type of non-life-threatening pain is that it's usually invisible. If somebody's experienced an obvious trauma – a car or bicycle crash, an operation, a surgical procedure – there is usually physical evidence of that trauma and pain we can all empathise with. Insidious-onset pain is, in effect, the opposite: instead of getting better as the weeks and months progress, it typically gets worse and forces us to modify our activities. In addition, it doesn't – at least not at first – prevent the patient from going about their daily life. Who hasn't battled their way into the office with sore knees, an aching back, a stiff neck, a slightly swollen joint? It is, we believe, to be expected: just part of having a body. But over time, the likelihood is that sore knee or stiff neck will worsen. Pain is incredibly difficult to describe but we can define acute pain as anything shorter than three months, after which it becomes chronic. And yet so much chronic pain appears slowly, gradually, and without a clear cause. Obviously, there are lifestyle factors that can increase the chances of such pain cropping up in the first place, but nonetheless for most doctors, physios and patients, pain without a prior injury or any 'source' is hard to comprehend. Sometimes, there just isn't any cause and effect.

The different branches of MSK therapy can be thought of as rooms – and together, they make a very large house indeed. We can work across intensive-care units, in cardiac rehabilitation facilities, in oncology, in gynaecology, in rheumatology. So many subsets to choose from – and some physios work across all of them. Across the course of my career, I've worked in both inpatient and outpatient clinics – the military, of course, being both hospital-based and across various rehab units. In many ways, the inpatient work is somewhat simpler. We can see, or at least trace, the root of a person's injury. We have notes, pages of them sometimes, that give us an indication as to what happened and why, what we need to do and when we can expect some results.

With insidious-onset pain, there's no such roadmap. People just turn up and explain that their back hurts, their knee or arm hurts – and they have no idea why. This would initially cause any physio to worry, especially those at the start of their career. What are we supposed to do with this information? We're trained to clinically gather information slowly, objectively, and decide on a plan of action, a roadmap, so to speak. The plan is then enacted. All of this is perfectly reasonable. But it's a lot of pressure when you're the one making the calls, giving the information and advice sheets and doing the actual MSK therapy sessions. The last thing you want is to make a patient's condition worse, which sadly will happen from time to time.

Every individual is different, too, so what works for one may not work for another. I can't say how each person's connections will differ or why. But I can guarantee they will. There's just so much information to take in when you sit down with a patient – either for the first or for the 100th time – and very little guidance as to how to process it all, how to decipher what you're hearing. At times it feels more like the job of a translator of some faraway, little-spoken language.

My work in the military enabled a wide spectrum of experiences to come my way. I was busy each and every day and becoming a more competent therapist every year – attending courses, educating myself as best I could. I realised that my work could positively impact someone who'd been in an accident or had surgery who needed some post-operative care, some MSK therapy as a result of a disease process which had badly affected their joints and or their soft tissues.

What does it mean to be ex-military? I started my working life in the Air Force as a Physical Education and rehab officer. I worked in the military for 16 years and served in two wars before leaving in 1992. I started in St Athan in 1976, then moved to Catterick, Halton, Bruggen and Queen Elizabeth Military Hospital, where I trained as a Remedial Gymnast. By this point, it was 1983, and I moved from being a PTI RG to a physiotherapist following a conversion course at RAF Halton

School of Physiotherapy. I then moved to Headley Court, to Chessington, to Gütersloh, to Cosford and to Brize Norton. This was to be my last posting, from 1990 to 1992.

Serving as a physical education officer was an excellent start for me. Troops get injured all the time, and it's so important that qualified medical personnel are available to help their recovery. The job is, as we know, an intensely physical one. We worked primarily on the musculoskeletal side of the body – the single most common reason for army personnel proving unfit to deploy or unable to fulfil their duties – but we also worked alongside officers, PTIs - Physical Training Instructors and Specialists to ensure they were aware of what needed to be done to avoid injury. Training can be brutal, but it needn't result in tears, sprains, breakages or similar. Back in the day, there used to be a prevailing attitude that 'pain equals gain' – something, thankfully, that is now being justly challenged and derided for the nonsense it is. No trainer wants his or her charge to get hurt – it won't make them stronger in any way, shape or form. I think I've been able to bring a lot of good into my current working practices as a result of my time in the RAF.

I reflect now on those early days when I was freshly qualified and had all that desire to learn and experience everything, and I feel a certain fondness for my younger self. What we're doing, essentially, is helping the body to work at its best, to move, to increase its potential. There's an awful lot of potential in our arms and legs, our torsos and abdomens, and untold untapped strength. But we do have to look after these bodies, these interconnected webs of muscle and sinew. I was attracted by the enormous amount of variety on offer – sporting teams, individual athletes, consultancy on musculoskeletal services, research for charities, private practice. The list was endless, it seemed, and every day, the physiotherapist is tasked with asking a series of questions and trying to puzzle out the answers.

So often, however, my patients came along to see me with very little information. They'd woken up one day with a pain, a problem, an ache that just refused to budge. It is incredibly hard to describe your pain to another human being: almost impossible, in fact. We can't put ourselves in the shoes of another, so we need to learn which questions to ask and how to interpret the answers. We need to watch the faces of our patients as we adjust an ankle, mobilise a knee or stretch out a calf. And it becomes even more difficult when we consider how much patients can over- or underestimate their pain. What is agony for one may be a slight niggle for another.

What we can agree on is the messaging: physical pain is associated with damage or pressure, which is building of one kind or another. This might be damage to a bone, a muscle, an area of tissue. It can be burning, stinging, throbbing, aching, sharp, dull, icy or hot. We each experience it differently, of course, but at its core, it's the only method our bodies have of alerting us to problems.

As the years went on and my experience grew, I realised something about insidious-onset pain. We might not have any idea what to do at the moment, and we just have to accept that. What we can do is ask questions. Instead of working from the top down, an approach favoured by many physios when trying to diagnose a problem, I realised that the system's central fulcrum is, in fact, the pelvis. There are three levers working from this central fulcrum: the trunk and two legs. It's the very centre, the pivot, a most important area. Unless there is an obvious problem, then my work becomes a process of moving up and down the chains, asking 'why' and trying to see if and how the problem can be cleared.

We learn a lot by moving slowly, by looking at a knee joint, for example, seeing how it responds, examining where something gets stuck, where a line is disrupted. A patient might be able to move more easily after physio, but does the joint or muscle or tendon actually move better? Does it work better? Is it playing its part appropriately as a part of the body's team?

I never made a conscious decision to focus my work on the pelvis as the preliminary point of investigation. My training didn't give me any grounding in this area; things gathered momentum in the 1990s – long after I'd qualified. Nonetheless, in the mid-'80s, I began to focus much more on this central area and to work with the lower limbs in a process of elimination. It made sense to me; it was logical. Since 1953, practitioners had been saying that the pelvis did not move, but as more and more work was done, it became clear that it did indeed admittedly, it is difficult to gauge how much it moves, but this hugely important factor would alter the process of so much recovery.

The three levers acting on the pelvis need to be able to work independently of each other, to dissociate their movements – between the cervical, the thorax, the lumbar spine, the hips, the knees, the ankles. So if a limb's orientation has changed, we look at the hips, knee and ankle, we ensure the pelvis is stable and look to see if the same is happening through the chains. It's much more widely accepted now that the pelvis moves, that it has the ability to enable load transfer up and down the chains. The pelvis is made up of large bones – there are the innominates, the sacrum together forming the sacroiliac joints posteriorly, and the symphysis pubis anteriorly the sacroiliac joints, are large L-shaped joints, shaped a bit like a propeller.

There are not flat surfaces here but smooth cartilaginous ones on the sacral side and a rougher cartilage on the other side, which causes friction. It is this change in the friction co-efficient at the joint that allows the increased load to be successfully transferred as this is the main role of the sacroiliac joints. We should not forget that the sacro iliac refers to the sacrum articulating with the ilium as opposed to the ilium articulating with the sacrum, known as ilio-sacral. The sacroiliac joints transfer load from the ground up, vertical ground reaction force (VGRF) and the top-down through gravity.

So we look at the torso, the legs, the head, the knees, the ankles and the feet: of course, we do. We want to make sure everything's working as it should. But first, I want to be sure that the pelvis is doing what it's intended to do – it has an influence, to a greater or lesser degree, on everything else in the body, even the diaphragm and the shoulder girdles. We notice very quickly when pressure has built up in this chain of connected tissues, nerves and muscles. Sometimes it's possible to see effects on the opposite side of the body to that described as painful; the body is three-dimensional. But all of this is used as information, evidence, clues to solving the problem. I would start with the pelvis with all types of pain and presentations, but it's particularly useful with insidious onset.

The RAF might have shaped me, but it's been the years – decades now – of elite sports MSK therapy that have really cemented my practice. I feel now that this approach is somewhat unique: a tried and tested method of addressing the many and varied problems these high-end elite clients and the general public bring to the table. And they're not just track and field clients but come from the whole range of sporting professions and disciplines. The most important thing, I think, is simplicity. Often, the best systems and the most efficient and effective are the simplest, the clearest. We need guidance and regulation: of course, we do. But we don't want to become algorithms/protocol-based, so at the core of our methods of working remains a simple principle: work with and look at the body and try to understand what it's doing. Easy, right?

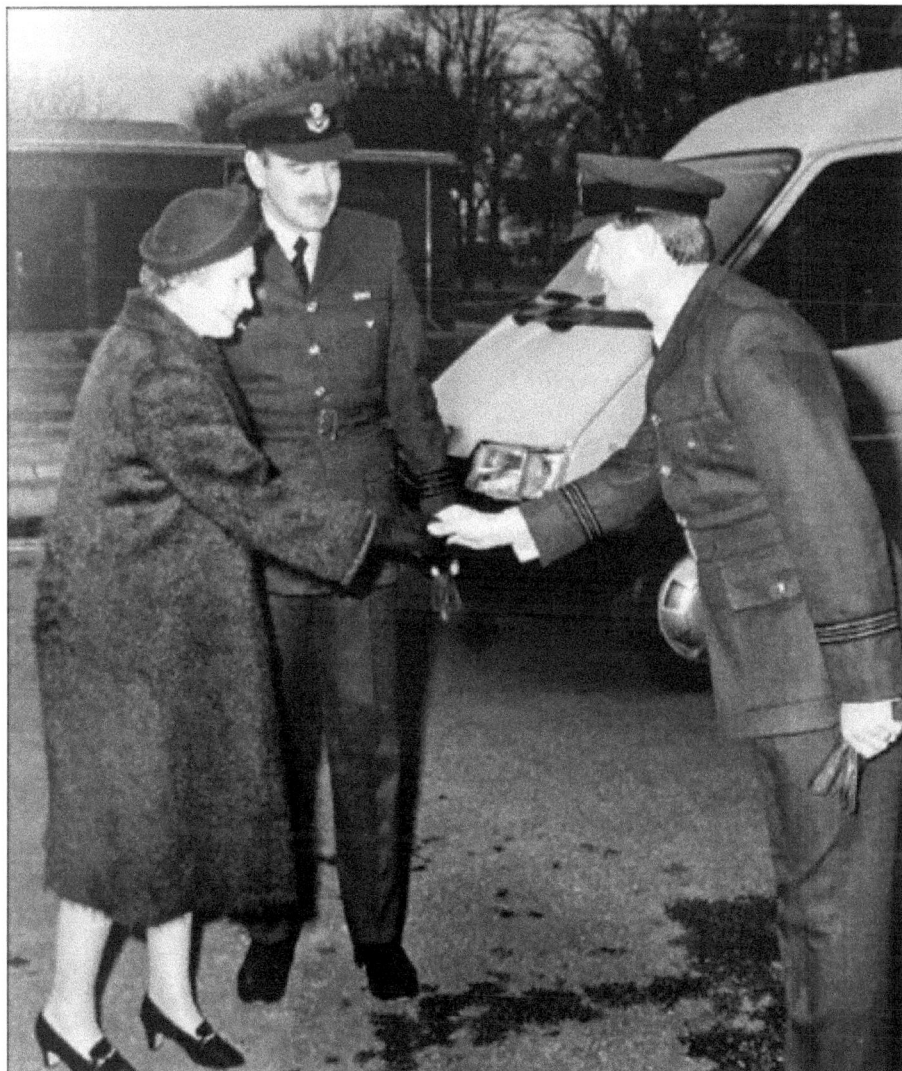

Meeting her Majesty Queen Elizabeth II when I was Officer Commanding Physical Education Flight at RAF Brize Norton 1991.

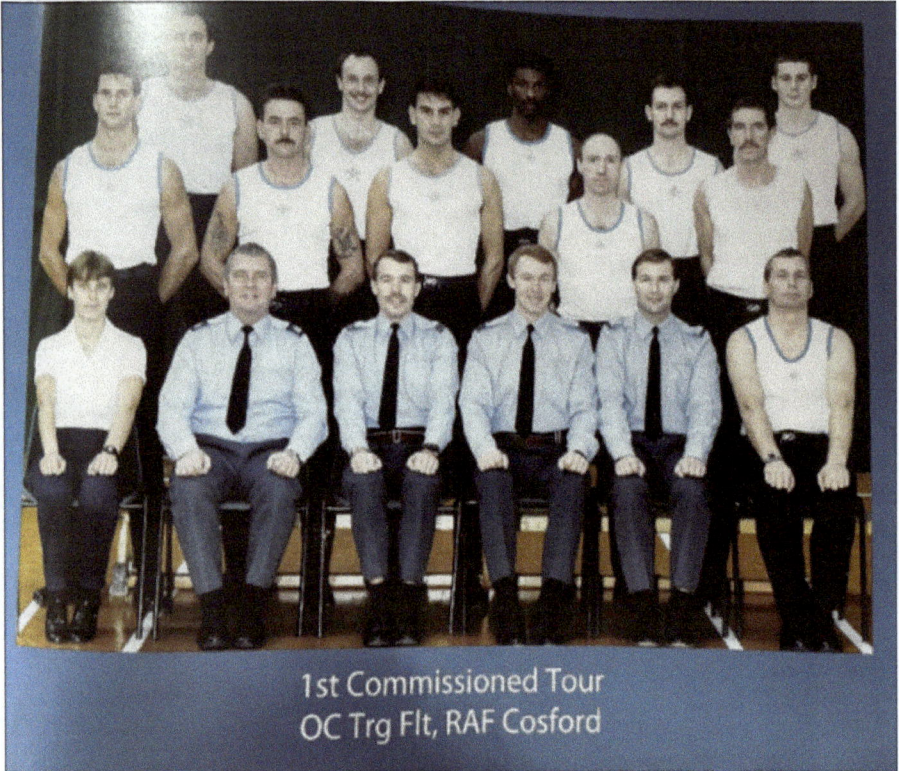

1st Commissioned Tour
OC Trg Flt, RAF Cosford

The RAF Cosford Physical Education and Training Team 1988.

3. A MEETING TO REMEMBER

In the mid-1940s, a young boy in war-torn Czechoslovakia began to experience a sore throat. Within a few days, this had developed into a headache, abdominal pain, aching muscles and a high fever. Within a week, he felt a little better – mostly. His legs continued to hurt a month later, and he experienced the occasional – bizarre – feeling of paralysis in one or both lower limbs. His calf muscles felt, if this was possible, somehow shorter, tighter, constricted. He noticed that his left foot seemed somewhat bent, curved in on itself, and attempting to uncurl it caused great pain.

If young Vladimir Janda had caught the virus just 20 years later, the consequences of his infection would have been minimal. Cases of polio dropped significantly following the roll-out of a successful vaccination programme, which has almost eradicated the illness around the world. Generally, polio is caused by contact with aerosol droplets passing from one infected person to another or from eating food or drinking water contaminated with infected faecal matter. Its insidious nature meant it could be spread from person to person without the infected victim having any idea they were ill; sometimes, it was weeks before symptoms developed. For many people, polio passes through the body's immune system, causing relatively little damage. But for the unfortunate few, long-term problems can persist for months and even years. Some patients are left with lifelong paralysis and deformity.

It is for this reason, among so many others, that MSK therapy is so important. It is likely that when Janda was a young adult, the options for rehabilitation were slim. He would have benefited, no doubt, from splints and braces, supports and occupational therapy. His joints, it appears, were certainly weakened by his infection, and though we don't know much else about how polio affected him, perhaps his career speaks for itself in that regard: perhaps the proof, as they say, is in the pudding.

It is largely accepted that Vladimir Janda pursued a medical career as a result of his experience with polio. Even in adulthood, he didn't have a huge amount of energy, and sometimes even standing up and moving around could be a chore. It must have been tough. I know he spent summers in Australia, benefiting from the ease of movement enabled by heat and the change in atmospheric pressure – he'd stay with another professor there; one can only imagine what it must have been like to be a fly on the wall listening to their conversations.

For me, the work of this man has been instrumental to guiding my own practice, and it is highly unlikely I'd be where I am today without his teachings and guidance. I am sure the work of Prof Dr Janda – a celebrated neurologist and lecturer – has inspired and influenced many thousands of people. He made enormous strides in the field of orthopaedic/neurological care. At its core, his philosophy focused on muscle imbalances and their interactions with the nervous system.

What was crucial, I think, was that – as is so often the case – Janda's physical 'shortcomings', if they can be termed as such, turned out to be his greatest strength. His skills in other areas seem to have been fine-tuned as a result: since large amounts of movement weren't possible for him, he needed to rely on the visual, and his acuity there was nothing short of remarkable. He'd ask patients to move so he could check one area or another, and soon enough he'd be able to see what was and what wasn't working. Since he knew how the body was meant to work, this was altogether easier – he joined the dots and linked so much of what was seen before as disparate. For me, he's the father of modern physical rehabilitation.

I'd been practising for 12 years when we met, and I was growing frustrated. In many ways, I met Dr Janda at the exact right time. It is so important, I realised afterwards, to have an industry mentor, to be able to connect with someone older and wiser and more experienced. You'd think over a decade in the business would count for a lot, and of course, it does – to an extent. But if you feel things are slowing down or not moving forward, or if your patients just aren't improving at the rate you'd like them to, then a certain amount of stress can set in.

There is nothing so dangerous in any job as boredom or the sense that your potential has already been fulfilled. Meeting Dr Janda showed me just how much I needed to learn, just how much was missing from my knowledge. I was never going to achieve my end goal – of helping more people – until I fundamentally changed the paradigm.

This is another point to consider: if I'd not attended the course, I'd never have had this 'Paul on the road to Damascus' moment. Young and older physios alike need to actively seek out industry experts and thinkers in order to broaden their horizons.

In the '80s, a lot of new work was being done on motor patterns: that is, how a muscle works within a team. Research on sequencing was being done, and though we knew things worked in a certain order, we didn't necessarily know at that time when a muscle should work in that team. What should come in first, second, third? Janda did a huge amount of work in this area and was one of the few advocating for this new way of thinking at the time. It was absolutely fascinating, and it resonated with me so loudly. His approach was direct, no-frills, no messing about. He seemed to really think about what he said and about the opinions he offered before he offered them, and he encouraged those he met in the industry to do the same. 'What are you trying to ask the body?' he'd say. 'Focus your mind.'

It's vital that any medical practitioner in any field should consider their words carefully. Patients are fine-tuned to pick up the slightest hesitation, the briefest of glances. The reason? They're in pain. Too many junior members of staff in hospitals and private facilities will posit theories in a stream-of-consciousness sort of way: 'Oh, it might be worth exploring the arthritis route. Or it could be a torn ligament. But the joint is weak, so it could also be repetitive strain. Is there any history of rheumatological problems in the family . . .?' and so on, until the patient's as confused as one might expect.

Janda was a breath of fresh air for the MSK therapy community at large. For so long, orthopaedists, as they were then known, focused on the specific area of the body in pain not necessarily what was causing the problem. As an example, a woman presenting with a painful right knee would be asked to demonstrate her ability to bend and stretch the joint, to possibly undergo an MRI, to have the joint examined and then potentially injected with anti-inflammatory steroids and muscle relaxants. This was known as the structural approach to pain management of the musculoskeletal system.

Now Janda argued something totally different, something previously unheard of. He suggested that chronic pain could not be treated simply by isolating the painful area or injury and ignoring the nervous system. It wasn't just the woman's knee that required attention when it hurt, but her whole motor system. It was not enough to see the problem in isolation – an island pain with nothing except water surrounding it.

Instead, the body as a whole needed to be taken into consideration: a cluster of islands, an archipelago – even a whole continent. It's all very well, he argued, to treat the woman's knee, to send her away with an exercise sheet, a structured timetable of exercises to complete each day, a raft of painkillers and a follow-up appointment. But perhaps it would be better to look for the cause of the injury, to assess where the body is weak and why the injury happened in the first place.

It was Janda who put forward the idea of two distinct groups of muscles: the tonic and the phasic. Tonic muscles cause the body to flex in on itself, and these develop while we're still in the womb, curled into the foetal position; phasic muscles are extensors – and these develop after birth. We use our flexors when we run, when we swim, when we walk. The name comes from the Latin verb *flexere*, to bend. And that's exactly what these muscles do: they decrease the angle between bones that meet at a joint. Think about what happens when you bring your knee up to your chest or up to meet the glutes for a standing quad stretch. Phasic muscles essentially work against gravity – they are prone to relax, in a nutshell. Though they're more dynamic than tonics, they are more susceptible to fatigue. While the tonics tighten, the phasics relax.

It was through observation and many, many trials with patients that Dr Janda developed his theories. He noted that after lesions occurred in the central nervous system, tonic muscles were spastic and sensitivity to the length of any stretching was increased, while the phasic muscles were utterly flaccid. It could therefore be extrapolated, he reasoned, that muscle imbalances were influenced by the central nervous system rather than coming as a result of structural changes in the muscles themselves.

And so it was that Dr Janda began a new form of Musculoskeletal-skeletal practice, one that rarely questioned patients' pain levels – as we noted in the previous chapter, these are so subjective anyway as to be almost useless. Instead, Janda went down a different route. The previously used structural approach was replaced by a more functional overall picture of the body's processes and systems. It did not focus on the single pathological area; instead, it adopted a more bird's-eye aerial view of a patient's condition when trying to address chronic musculoskeletal pain.

As such, Janda developed a series of tests to evaluate the movement of a patient. These were intended to identify muscle weakness and either confirm or rule out suspected causes of pain. The tests were:

1. Cervical flexion. Lying on their back, the patient is required to lift their head and look towards their feet. If the chin is raised first, the sternocleidomastoid muscle at the base of the neck is likely hyperactive and the deep neck flexor muscles weak.
2. Hip extension. The patient attempts, while lying on their back, to lift one leg. If activation of the glutes is delayed, the spinal muscles are tight and the abdominals weak.
3. Hip abduction. Lying on their side, the patient must lift their top leg and resist as the physio presses downward. If resistance is low, this suggests the core muscles are either weak or disengaged.
4. Trunk curl-up. The patient bends their knees to 90 degrees and places their heels in the physio's palms while lying on the floor. The patient curls upwards while maintaining pressure on the heels. If the pressure on the heels lessens early, the hip flexors are likely over-activated.
5. The push-up. Excessive elevation of the shoulder suggests that the scapular stabilisers are weak.

6. Shoulder abduction. This tests for cervical nerve compression
   or a herniated disc. While the patient sits down, they lift their
   shoulder, bend their elbow and place a hand on their head. If
   their pain is lessened, then it is likely they are suffering from
   cervical nerve compression.

Dr Janda's work, primarily, was about assessing patterns:
looking for clues and evidence that might suggest underlying
musculoskeletal issues that needed wholesale, rather than
specific, addressing. These patterns he categorised as Upper-
Crossed, Lower-Crossed and Layer Syndrome. These crossed
syndromes have gone on to play an enormous part in the
management of pain across the world. In essence, his theories
explain the specific muscle imbalances that patients
experience.

Upper Crossed Syndrome, or UCS, causes tightening of the
upper-body muscles and a chronic weakening of others.
These alternating zones create an X pattern. While the
pectoralis and levator scapulae tighten, the lower trapezius
and serratus anterior, for example, become weaker. Lower
Crossed Syndrome, or LCS, as the name suggests, causes
problems to the lower-body muscles – the tightening of the
rectus femoris, for example – and weakness in the abs and
glutes. Layer Syndrome comprises a combination of UCS and
LCS, and the patterns of weakness and tightness will
alternate. As might be expected, these patterns of tightness
and weakness create imbalances, and these imbalances, over
time, lead to compromised posture, injury and dysfunction in

movement. If left without proper care, these issues can result in joint degeneration. Essentially, then, the site of the patient's pain may not in fact be its cause.

At the time, Janda's approach was revolutionary. The idea that the musculoskeletal system and the central nervous system could be interdependent was novel. This sensorimotor system could experience one change that led, like a butterfly flapping its wings thousands of miles from the site of a hurricane, to a change in another part of the system. Ultimately our bodies strive for stability, homeostasis, but muscle imbalances indicate problems more often associated with neurological than structural change. It was Dr Janda who expounded the belief that patterns of imbalance were 'predictable' and that once initiated, they would spread throughout the muscular system.

When I was lucky enough to meet Dr Janda whilst attending a course in London on Myofascial Pain Syndromes, he introduced himself as a neurologist and a rehabilitation specialist. After the course, we started chatting, and before long, he had asked me several important questions. These were all related to the insidious-onset side of chronic pain and dysfunction, and they revealed to me just how much work I needed to do. It appeared I didn't know what the body was capable of in certain movement situations or how the body was meant to function when we moved – and if I didn't know that, how could I spot when the system was broken, when things weren't working? My only reference point would be pain and chasing the pain would not solve the problems of dysfunction.

This meeting with Dr Janda changed my life, and this is no exaggeration. If all I could rely upon were the verbal symptoms described by a patient, there was a very good chance I would not get to the bottom of the problem. I was finding that I just couldn't get there, to the root cause, to the central issue. Our training, all three years of it, was designed to cover everything – broad brush strokes, a huge church. And I completely appreciated the need for this; plus, no training is ever perfect by any stretch of the imagination. Nonetheless, I felt ill-prepared, especially for any sort of insidious-onset type issues – and I knew that if I felt this, many other therapists must be feeling the same. It wasn't that we weren't skilled or that we didn't have the knowledge or the talent. It's just that how it all came together was unclear until I met Janda.

I will say that training undertaken for all physios was far more hands-on back then. We used electrotherapy and focused much more on soft-tissue work. It was a tactile, incredibly practical course, and it couldn't have been more different to today's training programmes. I know that modern physios coming into the industry today are cut from a different sort of cloth: they are universally intelligent, especially since course requirements have altered, and they are now awarded a BSc instead of a graduate diploma. The amount of hands-on therapy has been substantially reduced, which – I feel – is a loss to the profession.

I could help deal with disease pathology, most post-operative issues or seronegative or seropositive spondarthritidies, and I could generally improve the quality of life of many patients, but I couldn't quite help get them right.

We can try and get our patients back to their pre-op levels of normality, or as close as humanly possible. When it came, however, to athletes or very active men and women who worked physically hard every day and whose bodies were beginning to complain – it felt like we as a profession, in my opinion, were hitting up against several glaring shortcomings. I was frustrated until I met Dr Janda, I think, without really knowing why. I knew that 30% of my patients would get better without any intervention whatsoever or even despite an intervention from me or any other colleague. In that regard there's always going to be a success rate of sorts. But I wanted to succeed with the other 70%, the trickier cases, the head-scratchers.

And sometimes, I realised, we were all making the assumption that because a patient's condition was improving, what we were doing and advising was working. It just wasn't the case, and I refused to kid myself about it. I'd see patients returning repeatedly with the same issues. It wasn't good enough. I wanted their function to improve, not just their pain. As I became more experienced and learned more, especially from Dr Janda and others, I began to realise that we can have very little direct influence on a patient's pain when it's of the insidious-onset variety. Instead, we can really try to improve their function. If this improves, their dysfunction will also improve and in turn their pain as well, especially if the dysfunction is the main reason for their pain.

I'm not sure what life, professionally, would have been like for me if I'd not met Janda. He asked me questions I should have been able to answer but couldn't. What happens, I thought to myself afterwards, when a body jumps or runs or walks? Not being able to answer, and having to give it some thought, was a useful experience in hindsight. I realised that I'd been putting sticking plasters on the problems of my patients.

I don't remember being trained to look at what the body was supposed to do – before injury, disease, operation. And because I didn't know that, I was not able to adequately assess when and how things went wrong. I needed to bridge the gap between what was happening and what was supposed to happen. And so, from that point, the objective was to develop methods to treat, mobilise and move while taking into account the whys and hows of a problem.

Janda was well-known for his work when I met him, but he could have published a lot more than he did. He was best regarded for his rehabilitation work: people speak of him as the master of rehab because he had this exceptional way of thinking outside the box. Indeed, some amazing tributes were written about him after his death.

I can remember wondering why he wasn't an international celebrity in the field, why he wasn't better known. Perhaps he resonated with me so strongly precisely because these methods of his weren't prolific, weren't the most highly praised. He was just so good when it came to chronic pain and why it was important to look at the history of a patient, to examine not just the injury but the whole picture. It wasn't about targeting one specific area in our work but about looking at everything.

There were others, too, of course, like the physical therapist Richard Dontigny and the PhD engineer Serge Gracovetsky, author of *The Spinal Engine*. Dr Andre Vleeming and his colleagues, who have written and compiled two volumes on *Low Back Pain the essential role of the Pelvis*, and Diane Lee, who helped interpret the work of Vleeming et al. Richard Dontigny did a lot of excellent work on the pelvis, how it moves and importantly, how it responds when loaded and offloaded. It wasn't until the late 1980s, early 1990s that the pelvic bone began to appear centre-stage at all. Before these two came along, nobody imagined that these enormous bones could move. Once it had been established that they could, it became clear that if it moves, it can go wrong.

The way that these people shaped new ideas in MSK therapy were pivotal moments. All physios will have one, I'm sure – a moment of epiphany, a moment when they realise that a particular method, figure or practice has ignited a renewed passion for the work. As a result, I began to seek out additional courses and books not just by Janda but by others like him. I felt buoyed up, empowered, ready to dedicate myself to learning as much as I possibly could. I was on the path to fresh insights that I would bring to bear on my own practice many years down the line.

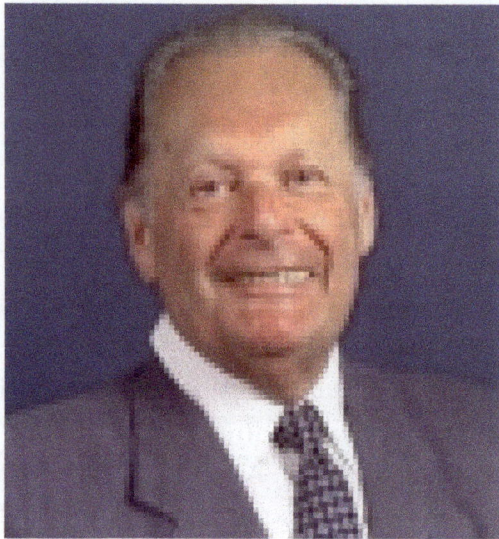

The late great Professor Dr Vladimir Janda, who single-handedly changed my thinking. Forever Grateful.

4. RELATIONSHIPS

It is clearly crucial, when examining an injury, not just to look at the area of pain. This was what I learned early on in my training, through Dr Janda, and it is a practice I have continued into the present day. And yet we also need to take the patient into account. We can only advocate for ourselves when it comes to pain: we can only say what hurts and how much, and we might decide in the moment to downplay the problem, over-emphasise one thing over another, underestimate how much the physio might be able to help. Humans come in so many different shapes and sizes, and it's crucial that we tailor any exercise programme or treatment plan to fit the expectations of individual patients.

So what is pain? This is a question many physios were trained to ask historically, but they didn't understand the answer. We need to respect that the patient has the pain – but if you follow the pain with insidious onset, you won't find the answer. Why not? Because first we have to find out why it's hurting.

Generally speaking, most MSK therapy practices offer an hour's assessment followed by 30 minutes of follow-up. I truly believe that more information is gathered in that first hour than anyone can possibly realise. These minutes allow us to accurately and clinically reason not only what we feel the problem is but also, more importantly, why this is the case. It's the 'why' that matters – more often than not, the 'what' is not too difficult by comparison.

With any patient, the MSK Therapist needs to be asking questions constantly. The body will respond – but we have to trust that it will. Questions need to be asked until they cannot be asked any more. I believe, in all honesty, that this is why, as a clinic, we have such a high success rate in terms of patient satisfaction. We follow that principle at all times. Experience counts for a lot in this game, that's for sure: what we all have is the ability to ask even the simplest-seeming questions, to take things back to basics. All too often, modern-day training relies upon a dogged acceptance of evidence-based pain, rather than its root causes. It's a sure-fire path to failure.

Clearly, understanding what a patient wants to get out of our time together is important. Once I know that, I can assess how likely I am to be able to deliver on these expectations. There are times, of course, when I will need to decide about the possibility of referring a patient to another service. If there are any red flags in that initial consultation, any physio discharging a duty of care to their patients will suggest that patient visit a sports-medicine doctor, their GP or an orthopaedic expert. Occasionally they will need to be sent for scans or further investigations elsewhere. This is a standard across the board.

It doesn't happen especially often anymore, particularly with any sort of musculoskeletal problem, but from time to time I will of course ask someone on my team to sit in during a consultation, just to be sure nothing's being missed and we're on target. One patient of mine has been attending consultations for two years, and it's only recently that we've started to notice some progress in her condition. This is not, of course, a frequent occurrence, but it's certainly true that once someone comes to see us at the clinic, they've usually been around the houses somewhat already. We really underestimate just how much people are bumped around the system, how frequently they're passed from one department to another.

It's a constant process of assessment. And it's not an easy one by any stretch: in layman's terms, the human body contains about 600 muscles, which can be divided into three categories: skeletal, smooth and cardiac. They usually work in a team – one set relaxing, the other tightening – and though most do both, some other muscles will be stabilizing, some will be stopping the unwanted movement of the prime mover. This is known as "group-action of muscles". These first principles are crucial to understanding the beginnings of sequences: how something works and why. Muscles also work in teams to produce a smooth coordinated movement.

We must return to the work of a physiotherapist and how it is in many ways similar to that of a detective. All of our assessments take into account not just the reports of pain and an observation of the affected area but also the patient's history, their lifestyle, the cause of their pain as they see it.

Take for example a patient of mine – Mrs Jones – who complains of shoulder pain. She's seen her consultant about it three times, had some local therapy and received some steroid injections. Nothing much seems to be working, and she's had this problem now for 18 months. We sit down together.

'So is there anything else that's been causing trouble?' I might ask.

'Well, my right ankle plays up occasionally. It was a while ago, and it was hurting really badly – but then it seemed to get better.'

In not much time at all, it becomes clearer that the right ankle never really recovered from whatever happened to it: the body simply adapted. We all bear an enormous load every day – we move these loads via joint and fascial systems throughout the body. In this case, from the right ankle through to the left shoulder, and this was the reason the chain was no longer working. This is due to both mechanical and fascial changes. If one aspect of that chain isn't working, the whole system is under pressure. And we're designed to move, so we do so, and the chain tightens and stiffens – this can all happen without us feeling a single bit of pain. Remember the body has a few options available when it is not functioning optimally – it can tighten, stiffen and the become painful and the more we ignore it the more it increases these defence mechanisms.

It should be the aim of every physio to treat the patient, not the condition. It isn't our job to decide what's relevant and what isn't. During every hour-long first appointment, a patient and I will spend a good 40 minutes discussing them and their life. I need the history, and I need to be able to narrow down the wide span of possibilities. The more they talk about themselves and their lifestyles and environment, we can get a better picture of what their body is doing. Think, just for a moment, about all the myriad things that can, potentially, cause problems in the body. That first appointment is crucial – it's like being a magpie, gathering the treasure, which is someone's ability to explain what's happening. Once they've done that, they can leave the information with their physio.

What is fascinating, I think, is just how much society has changed in the past century. People used to be accustomed to waiting, to taking their time: they queued for rations and coupons during the war; they queued to send telegrams or letters that took weeks to arrive; they stood in line patiently in the first weeks of the NHS as appointments began to be filled. Our present culture has ensured the new generations have a different attitude, I think. We now live in a world of rolling news coverage, refreshed social-media feeds, Amazon Prime and 24-hour delivery. If we want something, we want it yesterday.

Contrast this, for a moment, with the time it takes the average person to secure an NHS appointment. GPs and physios on the Health Service can usually provide between 10 and 20 minutes, if that, to their patients. There is no time for any conversation about past symptoms or recovery from injuries: the main necessity is to firefight, to ensure that the needs of the present day – the here and now – are being met, to send the patient away with a checklist and a prescription. The way that private physio practices work does the opposite – we're not trying to simply solve the problem as it presents on the day in question. The NHS is a superb service for in-the-moment primary care, but I think for anyone with more chronic problems, a more holistic, all-round approach is required. Private clinics simply have more time, and this is the crux of the difference between the two.

Another patient – let's call him Mr Thompson – comes in for a problem with his hip.

'Anything else?' we ask.

'Oh no, just the hip.' He pauses. 'Well, actually, now you mention it – my elbow's been a bit stiff recently.'

This is an example of a patient advocating for a part of their body. The patient knows more about their body than we do. If they mention it, their body feels it's worth mentioning. Think about it – there's a reason they bring it up, right? And of course, the hip and elbow may not be linked at all. But they may be completely connected: we just need the information, all of it, in order to proceed with a plan.

Treatment is the easy part, really, once we know what we're trying to achieve. I also see treatment not as the answer but a physical question. The body is complex, and I can't possibly know as much about a person's body from an hour's consultation but then again, I don't have to, the body knows the answers – I just need to know what questions to ask.

I feel strongly that my team should treat their own patients however they see fit: when I teach or provide training courses, I'm not trying to put them on my journey or pathway, simply to help them join the dots better. We've all completed the same training; we all started in the same place. What's really fascinating, for me, is how often a patient will reference a historic injury – 'I had a problem with my big toe 10 years ago,' for example – and then mention how it just 'went away'. In reality, of course, the body simply adapted to whatever new stance was required of it.

As human beings we're not a science, there is science within many aspects of the way we function but as a whole science does not explain all that is needed, we require pragmatic and anecdotal input; so yes, the art. The body moves throughout the course of our lives until the day it doesn't any more. Our bodies slow down over time even though we might not realise it: the niggles and pains that caused few problems at 21 become more pronounced at 30 and again more so at 40. We might not feel any pain at all in the left knee until we play a certain sport for more than 40 minutes or run a longer distance than usual or do backstroke in the swimming pool rather than front crawl.

We know there is the maxim 'if you don't use it you will lose it', pertaining to the body and we all become more linear in our movements and tend to repeat the same patterns as we get older. There is no exact algorithm or equation to work out why the body does what it does or why it reacts in certain ways. All we can do is ask questions of it and see what responses come back. Shockingly, there is no research on the "normal" state of the body after the age of 65. Therefore, we've no academic evidence beyond our own experience of how a body might be reacting at 70, 80 or 90.

One of the frustrations, occasionally, is nothing to do with patients themselves but with medical information passages. The left hand never seems to know what the right hand is doing: something that really does need to change, especially as populations get older and it becomes more important than ever to ensure efficient communication systems. Think how difficult it is to move from one county to another, for instance, and effectively 'bring' your medical records with you. The different counties and systems, the public and private, don't speak to each other. And so, inevitably, things are missed. This can be very frustrating for patients, who, especially when in pain, need their medical care to be cohesively examined, joined-up and well-organised. We might have fewer patients presenting with chronic issues if these two sectors communicated more effectively.

Too often, patients in pain are dismissed. If the pain's source isn't obvious, either to private or state medical practitioners, they are escalated up the ladder to various different specialists who might not have any real answers for them. Indeed, sometimes they're even made out to be crazy. The most important thing as medical professionals and for us as physios is to listen.

And we also need to understand the person in front of us – their age, education and background. We need to see and assess very quickly how best to communicate with them. It often feels as though our work relies on an element of intuition, on being able to read a room or situation very quickly and effectively, on the ability to look beyond what a patient is telling us.

As a physio, it is vital to examine a patient's internal and external environment. If a person lives in a high-rise building with no access to a lift, for instance, I might reasonably assume their injuries – whatever they present with – might be exacerbated by frequent walks up and down many flights of steps. Similarly, they might casually mention that they swim four times a week at the last moment during our consultation, making a previously puzzling injury suddenly much more understandable.

External environments can be anything from where in the country a person lives to their home's proximity to the sea, a main road or their doctor's surgery. It can comprise their access to technology – whether they have a computer or WiFi at home, whether they use the internet and how often, whether they use their computers primarily for work eight hours a day or for 20 minutes of web-browsing in the evening. How often does this patient see their friends, partner, family? How often do they travel abroad, and what do they do when they get there? How well is the workstation they use fitted to them and do the facilities they frequent allow for there their height or weight. Do they have space to move around easily at work or at home?

Internal environments are different. These comprise a person's lifestyle: their exercise routines, their alcohol intake, their consumption of sugar, whether they smoke or take recreational drugs, whether they spend their weekends partying or lying on the sofa. What is their walking gait like, do they have arthritic changes at the joints? Is there obvious muscle atrophy or a greater muscle bulk in different areas of the body affecting their function? As we speak during these initial consultations and those that follow afterwards, a picture begins to come into focus, a portrait we can add to as we go along the journey. The key thing is to listen.

A patient comes to see me – a young female athlete studying a PhD alongside her training. She's focused, hard-working and disciplined: like all athletes, she has to be. She's a middle-distance runner, placing consistently highly across 1500m, 3000m and 5000m races and cross country – these races can take place anywhere in the country or overseas, so travel time is an example of external environment, another factor in an already busy life.

She came to see me in late 2021, we've been working together for some time already. She travels from quite far away – no small distance when our appointment's at 10am. She's been struggling with her hips, right more than left, pain for some weeks now, a pain that begins just minutes after she starts training.

'I can still train,' she says, 'but not to the same degree.'

There are a number of questions I need to ask in order to establish the mechanism of the injury and why her hips are reacting as they have been. We need to understand the 'why' as the what is fairly obvious. The patient in front of you will have most of the answers but you need to spend time working through the whys. We discuss whether the hip feels tight or sore immediately after she's finished working out, how fast the pain comes on during her training and non-training days, what does her preparation look like before and after training and whether the tension changes after 24 hours or less.

'The pain starts on the bone,' she tells me, pointing to the greater trochanter, 'and the day after the run I'll do loads of stretching, and that doesn't feel great. It usually feels a bit better the day after.'

I'll record these responses as they're speaking, but all the while I'm thinking, *what could be causing this reaction? What's the mechanism and where do I need to look to influence the mechanism?* Clearly, I have not examined her yet but the physical examination becomes easier if you have some ideas around the mechanism to help determine the best method of trying to help her. The problem is going to become cumulative given she has been struggling for a few months and continued to train, so clearly whatever has caused this issue is one thing, but it has been compounded by the amount of strain put on the tissues, so we will need to manage her painful site whilst understanding the mechanism, the 'why'.

I'll say it again: if you don't know what is supposed to happen, how do you know when it's not happening?

In these situations, you invariably end up treating the symptoms and not the cause. I am not suggesting that the symptoms don't require some management, but you must be careful not to pacify the symptoms and think it's all good. Experience has taught me the symptoms will return and the body will have further adapted, making the whole situation worse...

When starting the physical examination, I need to establish how she is loading in stance, is the weight felt easily through both legs and is it more towards the heels or the toes, does she stand with her legs wide apart or under her shoulders? Is there any obvious rotation at the spine/pelvis? Is there any change to the shoulder positions or the neck/head position, assuming I know what her normal pain-free and fully functioning start point is?

I then need to see how she is moving at the spine, pelvis and hips to see if they are coordinating and importantly do they dissociate? Where does she initiate each movement from and what is the quality of the movement? Range is important but not as much as the quality in my opinion. The quality of movement can be described as the acceleration and deceleration about the joint: the smoother the movement the better the quality. The laws of mechanics state that once movement about a joint is reduced in one plain, then all other plains are reduced, and this can have a long-term effect on flexibility and function. Over the next 40 minutes, I try to help the joint function better, to increase the ease and quality of movement, and this, in turn, will improve the available range. Once we have increased the range it is important to re-establish control about that joint and the associated structures. *Remember we train movement, not muscle!*

Athletes have been to see me many times over the years. They could easily book in with a physio closer to home, in the capital, but they are also aware that there are a huge range of abilities and specialties and that once they have found someone who knows and understands how their musculoskeletal system works, it's better not to upset the apple cart by going elsewhere. 'I was trying to find someone specifically to help with my soft tissue,' the athlete I'm seeing says, as we work through a range of exercises.

I know that to treat athletes, I can't see her as 'normal'. She trains five days a week: two interval sessions, one longer run and a maximum of five hours' cross training a week – usually swimming or cycling. She's doing around an hour to 1.5 hours of exercise every day, putting her body under an enormous amount of pressure. And she's not even a full-time athlete, remember – somehow, she needs to find the time to do all this work, to put in all this effort, alongside her studies, not to mention her everyday life. It's the mental fatigue that can prove problematic for many athletes, quite apart from the physical. There's so much going on for her, and she's functioning at a consistently high level.

The thing about energy, I know, is that once an athlete – once anyone – has drained their cup, it really is empty. We're human beings and we get tired. We need therefore to understand how much an athlete – or any client – is adapting and modifying their life to compensate for an injury, how much their fatigue might be contributing to the problem not getting better. Our bodies are designed to be efficient, and this efficiency gives us the ability to function at a higher level for longer. However, we can still be effective but not necessarily efficient. Athletes in particular understand that the body will occasionally say 'enough'; it's how they respond to it that really matters. It's all too easy for someone to become fed up when an area they've given time and attention to, a part of them they've advocated for, isn't improving. But it's our job to try and see what the real problem is, why is there a problem and, whether it's indicative of something else.

Whenever we see a client, we know that we need to examine all the factors contributing to their injury and in particular we need to understand the mechanism: there it is again, the mechanism, not just the injury itself. And when we prescribe a treatment plan, a way of moving forward, of maintaining as much function as possible without hindering the healing process, we need to be able to justify our view; our clinical or critical reasoning, take in all the elements and then explain how we're moving forward. It's that explanation, perhaps more than anything else, that clients need and appreciate. I will come on, later, to the problems associated with human beings – to the myriad things that can and often do go wrong. That's to be expected. As with all my clients, it's how we respond as physios to the information we have gathered that can make all the difference.

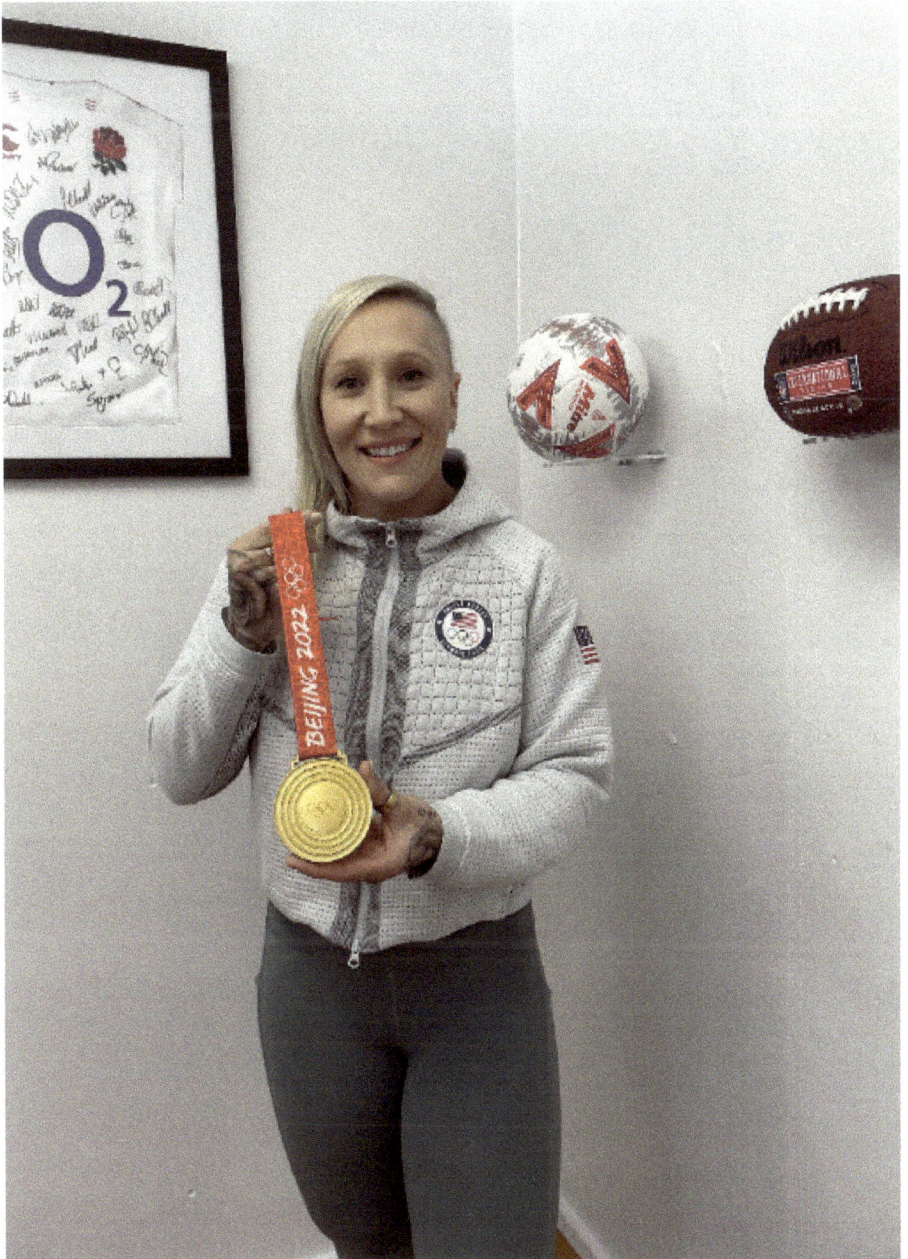

Kaillie Humphries four-time Olympic Champion, five-time World Champion Bobsleigh, still competing. Keeps me on my toes!

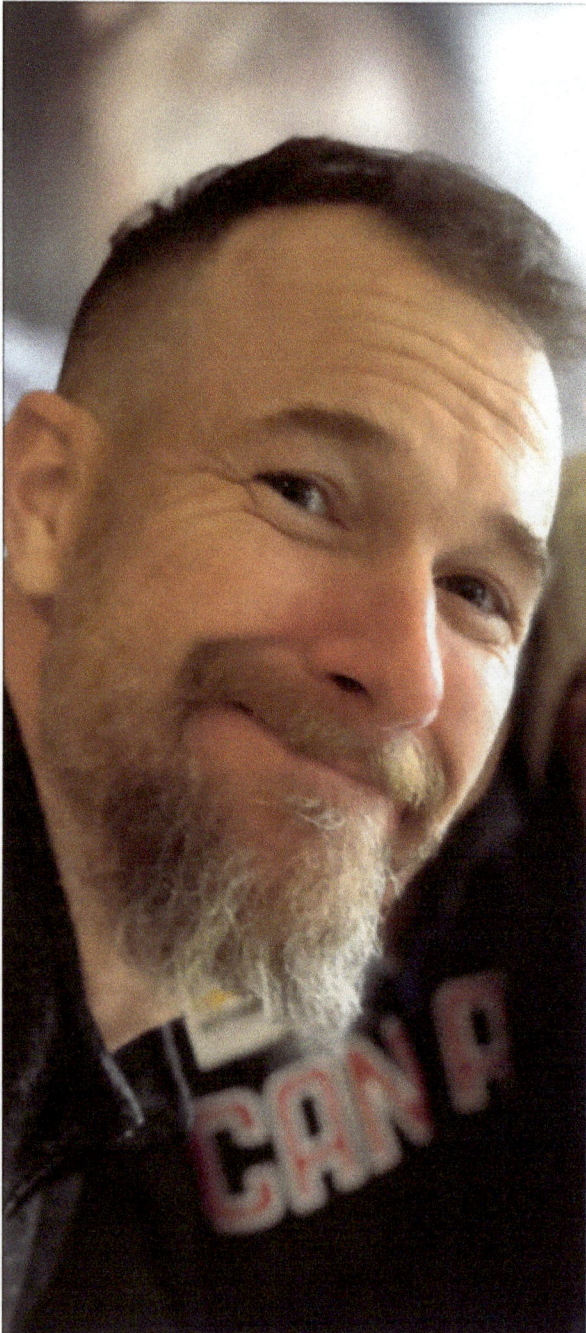

A rare smiling photo of my friend Stu McMillan, great sprints and Bobsleigh Push Coach. We met in the Canada in 1995.

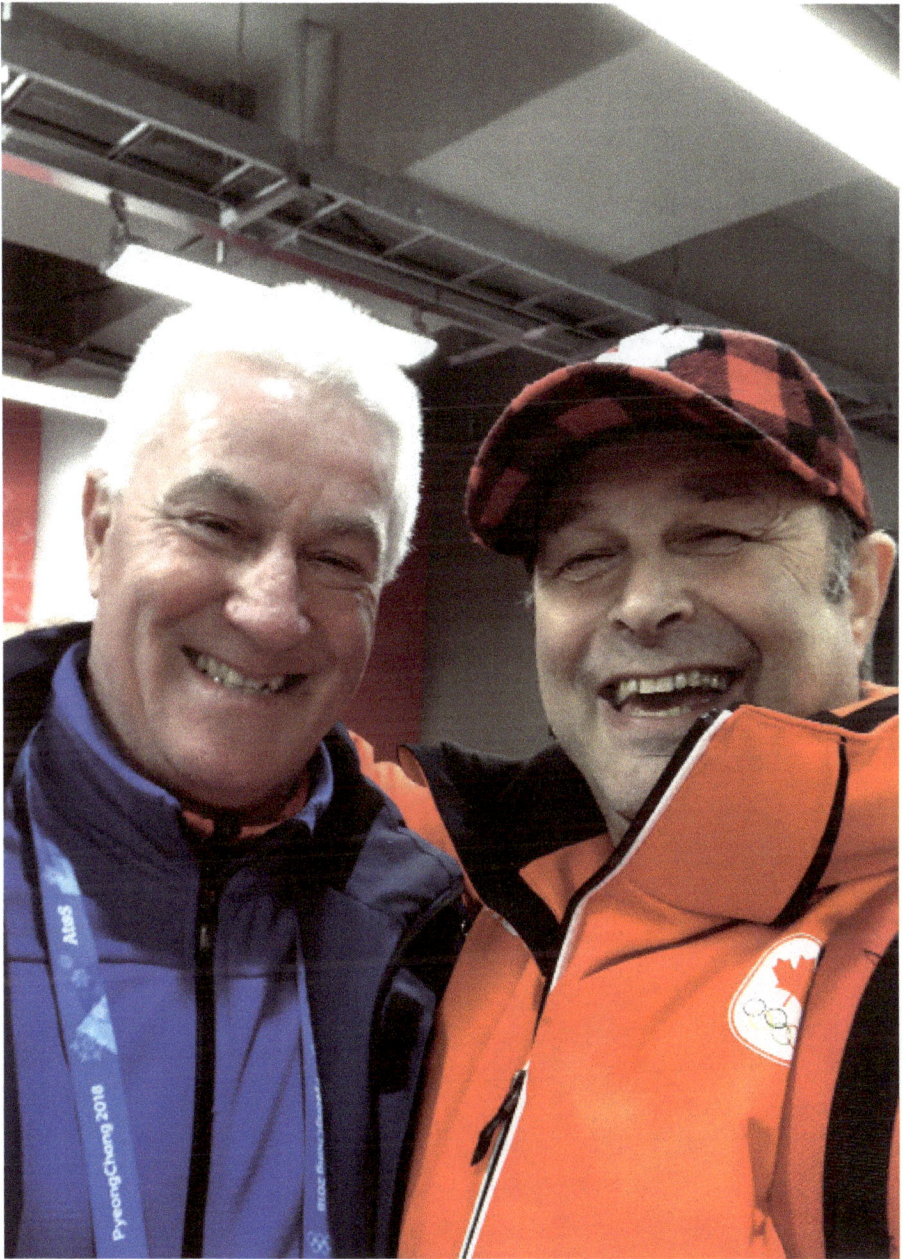

Tom De La Hunty my long standing best friend and Multi National Bobsleigh Coach
who was an excellent Driver learnt a lot

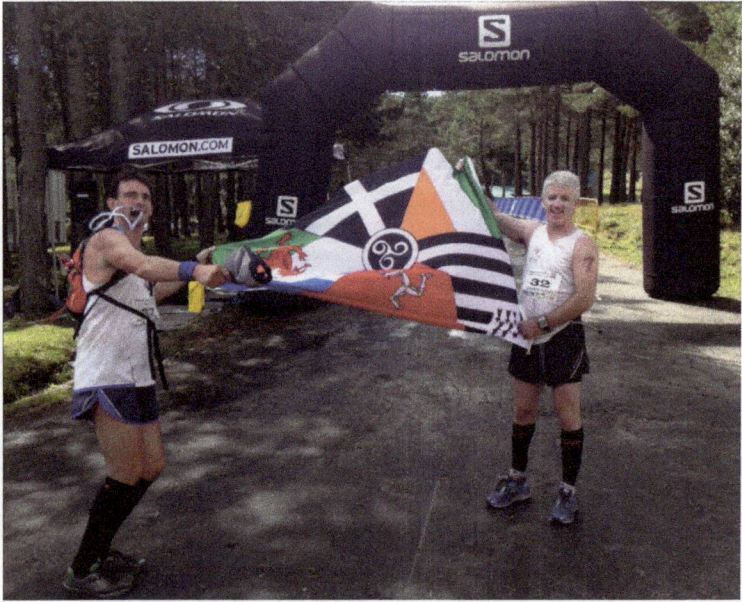

Crazy French Chef Stephane Delourme and an Irish Financial Wizard Peter McGahan ran the 7 Celtic Marathons.

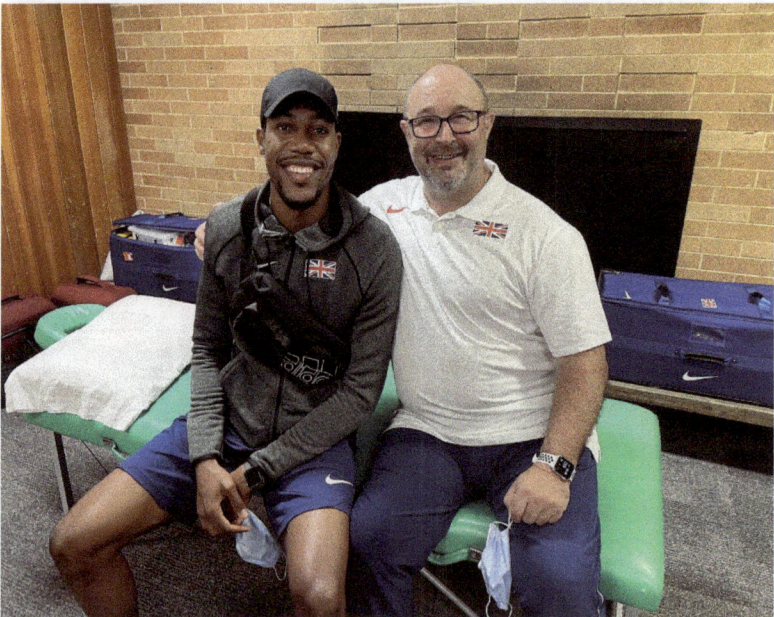

Zharnel Hughes sprinter, World Medalist 100m 2022 and 2023 and Pilot.

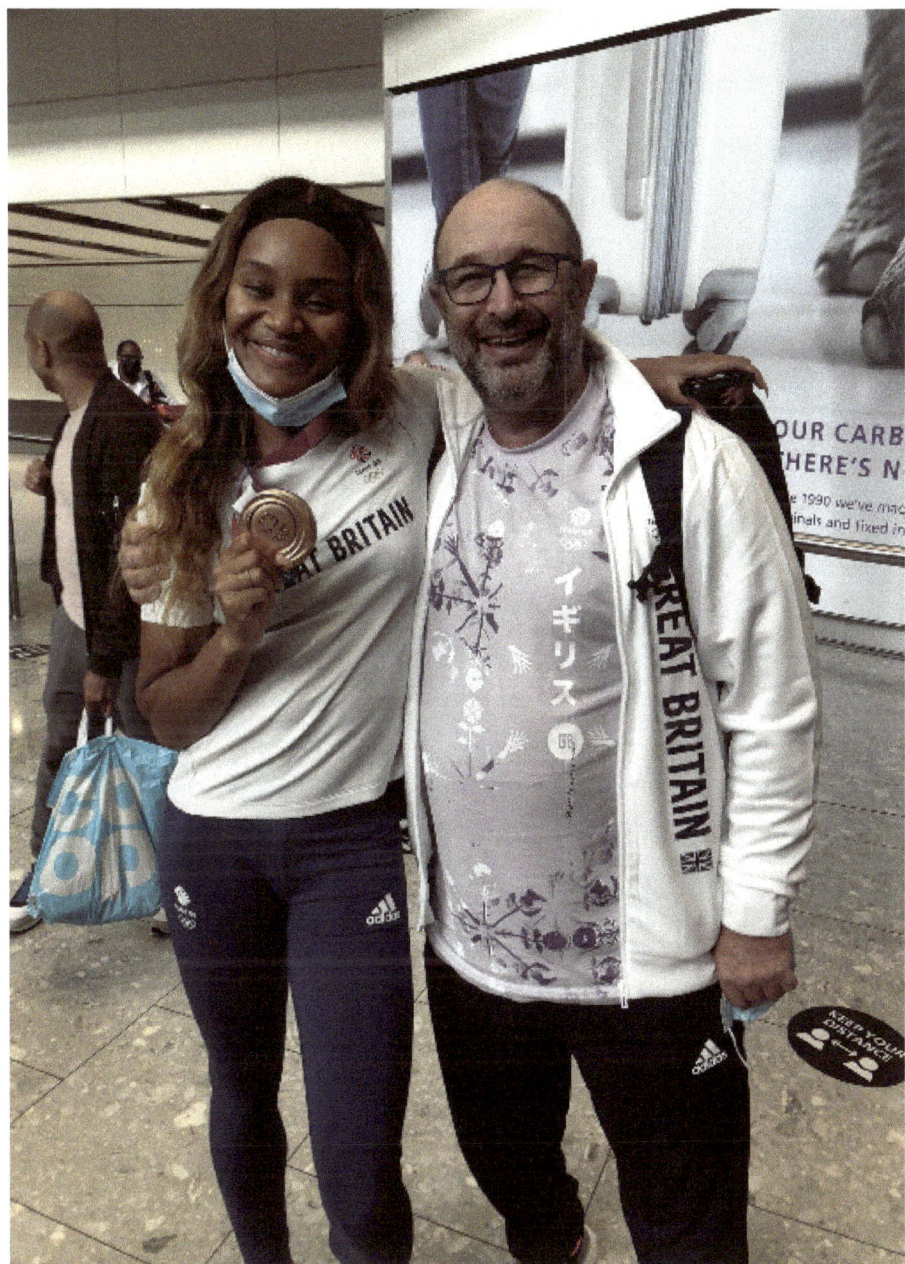

Imani Lara Lansiquot, 100m Sprinter Olympic and World Relay Medalist, Nike Athlete. We work together.

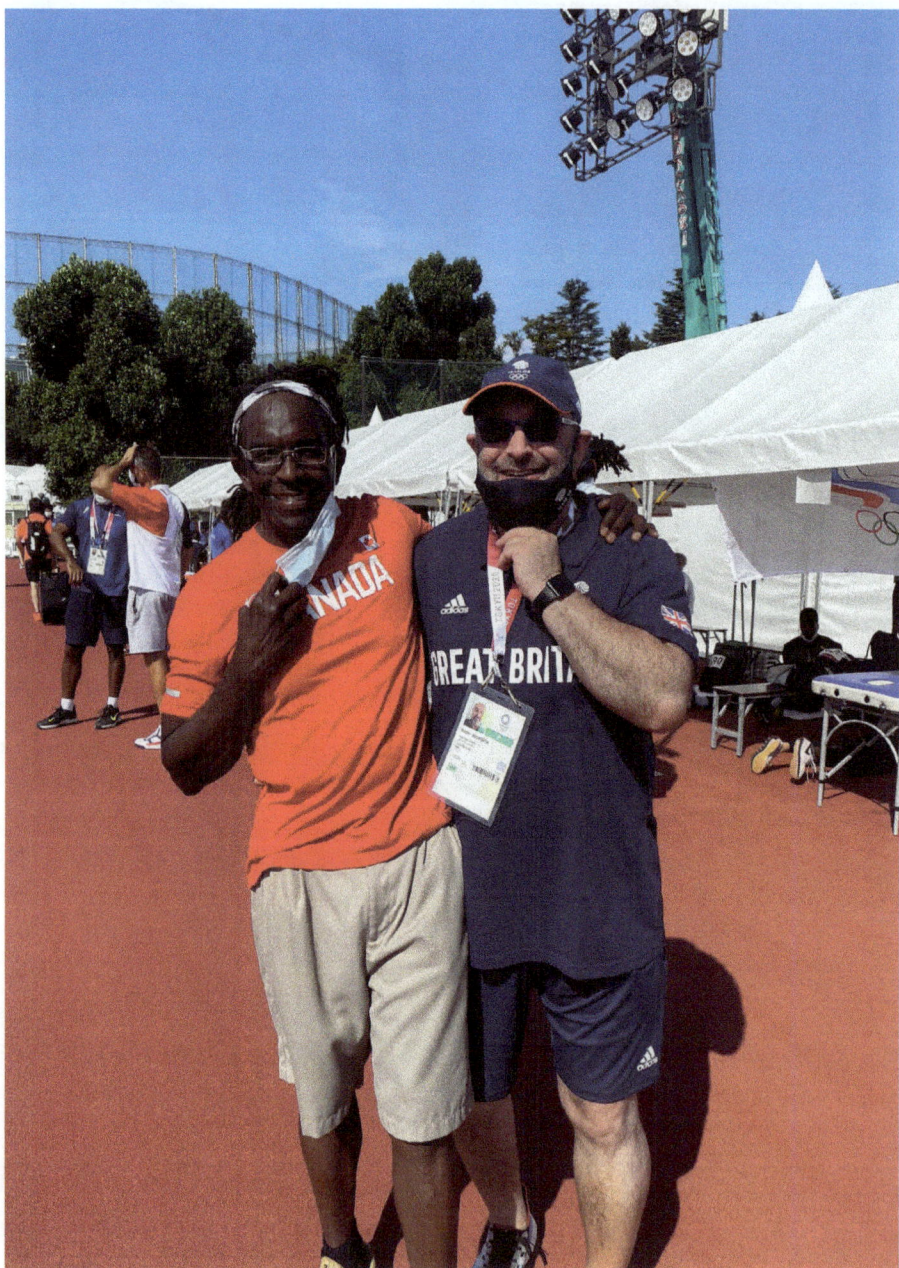

My very good friend and colleague Wilbur, we met in 1998 on a mountain with athletes.

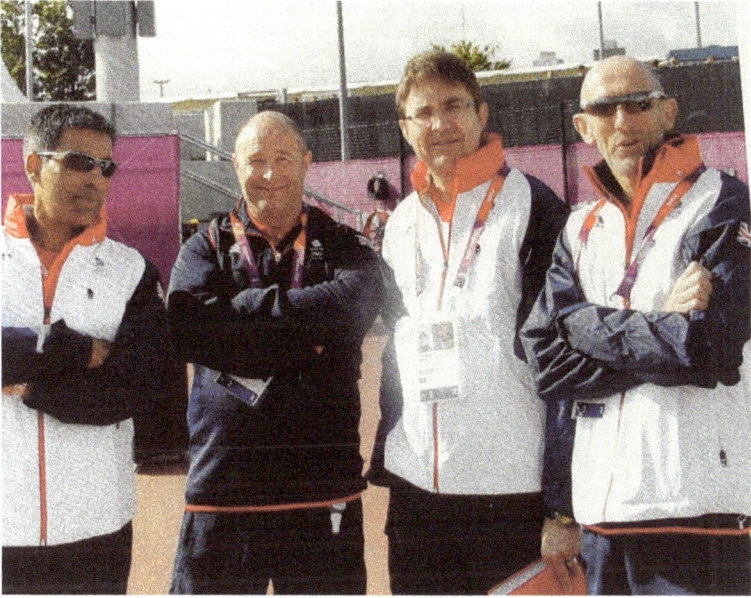

London 2012 - Dr Rob Chakraverty (MO), Dr Paul Dijkstra (CMO) and the late Neil Black, Head and Science and Medicine.

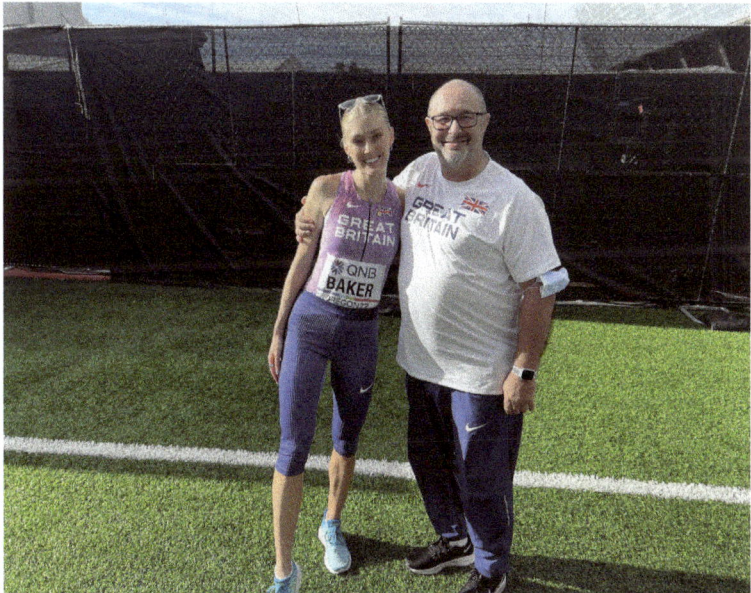

Ellie, like all middle distance athletes, works hard and as result needs help. So I do my best!

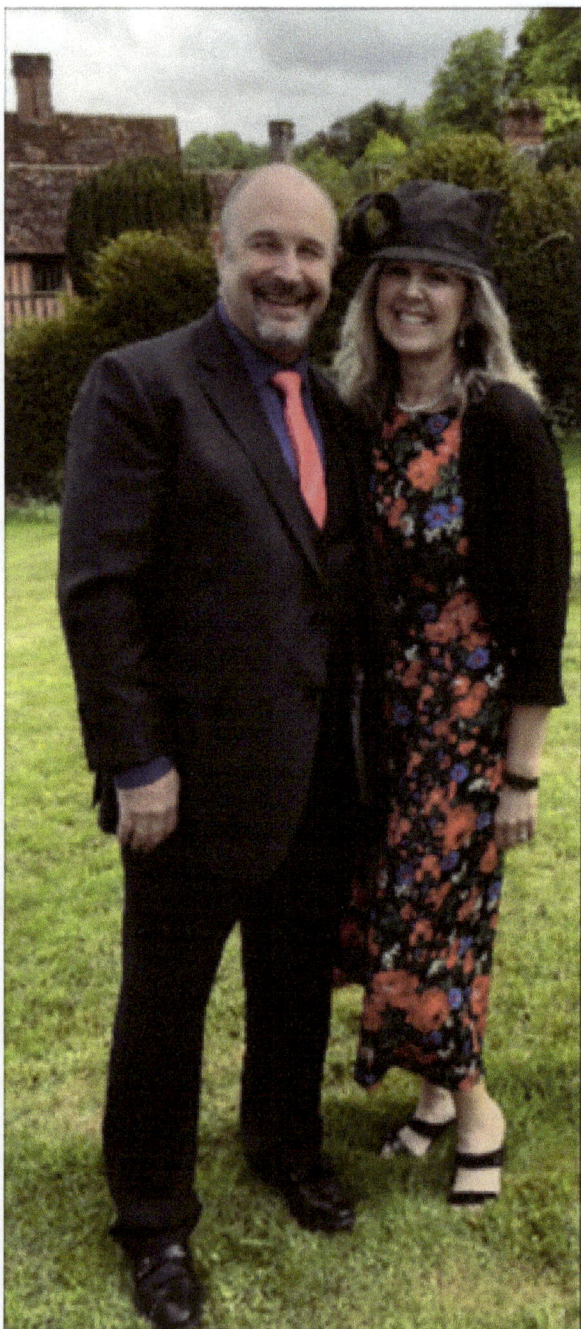

It wouldn't be right not to have a picture of the most important relationship in my life, Kim.

5. PUBLIC AND PRIVATE

A little bit of history... by the first year of the so-called Great War, a troupe of massage therapists had been trained to work at British military hospitals. They'd begin at 9am and see between 30 and 40 patients a day. Their treatments ranged from massage to hydrotherapy, electrotherapy, ionization, and radiant heat. It was one of the first times that alternative forms of medical attention were recognised as beneficial in a more wholesale, generalist environment. Physios were known back then as masseurs, and they fell under the branch of 'nursing'. By 1894, the Society of Trained Masseuses was founded by four nurses.

By the time the Second World War began, physiotherapists had become highly sought after; the polio epidemics of the time had resulted in many people, especially children, requiring long-term muscular rehabilitation. Added to this, of course, were the many hundreds of wounded soldiers returning home and requiring intense regimes to help them heal. As is so often the case, demand was rising for this particular, specialised form of treatment – and as such, over time, the reputation of physios was gradually improving.

Towards the end of that war, the Society changed its name: it was now the Chartered Society of Physiotherapy. The profession was still regarded rather dimly by doctors, who often directed them in public hospitals. Most treatments revolved around massage and exercise, as well as water-based therapy for the treatment of joint and nerve injuries. The problem, of course, was facilities – few field hospitals had the money or space for hydrotherapy pools, and makeshift baths were often used instead.

By the 1950s, physios were granted licence to manipulate the spine and extremity joints. They also began to move out of hospitals and into schools, rehab centres and outpatient clinics. The '50s and '60s saw a surge in the recognition of MSK therapy. This was largely a result of the Professions Supplementary to Medicine Act, which resulted in State Registration. Prior to this time, any practitioner outside the traditional medical realm had the option of registering voluntarily under the Board of Registration of Medical Auxiliaries. Here one might find so-called 'speech' therapists, opticians, radiographers, chiropodists, dieticians, physiotherapists, and orthotists. It was the British Medical Association who kept an eye on all these different branches, ensuring that employees were treated fairly and trying to improve their status in the medical community and, by extension, their working conditions and pay.

By 1968, when the Central Health Services Council set up a sub-committee on rehabilitation, the aim was to 'consider the future provision of rehabilitation services in the NHS, their organisation and development, and to make recommendations'. Every member of the committee – 16 people – were doctors, but not one speech therapist, chiropodist or physiotherapist was present. Not a single member of the so-called 'remedial professions', as they were known back then, was invited. Their aim was to consider occupational therapy, remedial gymnasts and MSK therapy across the NHS and assess their relations among the different branches with regards to rehabilitation.

The consultant will have overall managerial responsibility for the rehabilitation services and will decide how the general day-to-day running of the rehabilitation should be organised according to local circumstances. We recommend that delegation of responsibility for day-to-day treatment of patients should be permitted to members of the remedial professions, provided that they are always under the supervision of the appropriate consultant. (DHSS 1972)

Nonetheless, some key findings from the report do stand out:

While the doctor must retain responsibility for the patient and for the prescription of treatment, more scope could and should be given to the therapist in the application and duration of treatment prescribed . . . many physiotherapists feel obliged to give treatment they consider to be inadequate and ineffective, either because the treatments are not sufficiently intensive, or because they are primarily palliative. (DHSS 1972)

It was clear that more representation of these professions was required, particularly at regional levels across the country. Physiotherapists and their counterparts needed to be involved in decision-making and policy creation and their expertise taken into account when treating patients. In addition, it was recommended that a career structure be put in place to enable senior posts with clinical, research and teaching responsibilities.

On the whole, this report certainly did more harm than good in the sense that it reconfirmed what many outside the physio and other similar professions already felt. The dominance of so-called 'traditional' medicine was re-established, and yet, it's not all black and white. Career progression and research, representation and treatment-plan authority were all mentioned, mostly because committee representatives from the 'remedials' insisted on their inclusion in the statement.

The UK is rightly proud of its NHS, particularly so over the tumultuous Covid period. There is an awful lot of good feeling about the system and its staff – it is ranked, consistently, as one of the things British people feel most proud of. And yet, if I'm honest, I see it as a pilot scheme. The will to succeed is extremely high and always has been. But very little has changed since the service's inception in 1948, when society – as we know – was different in almost every regard.

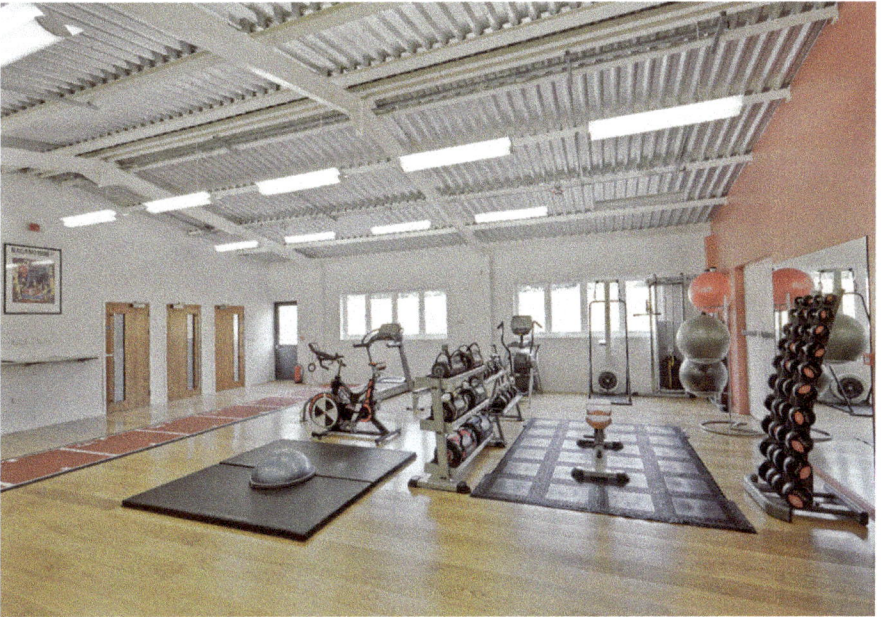

The rehab facility at the clinic is fully equipped and available to all patients.

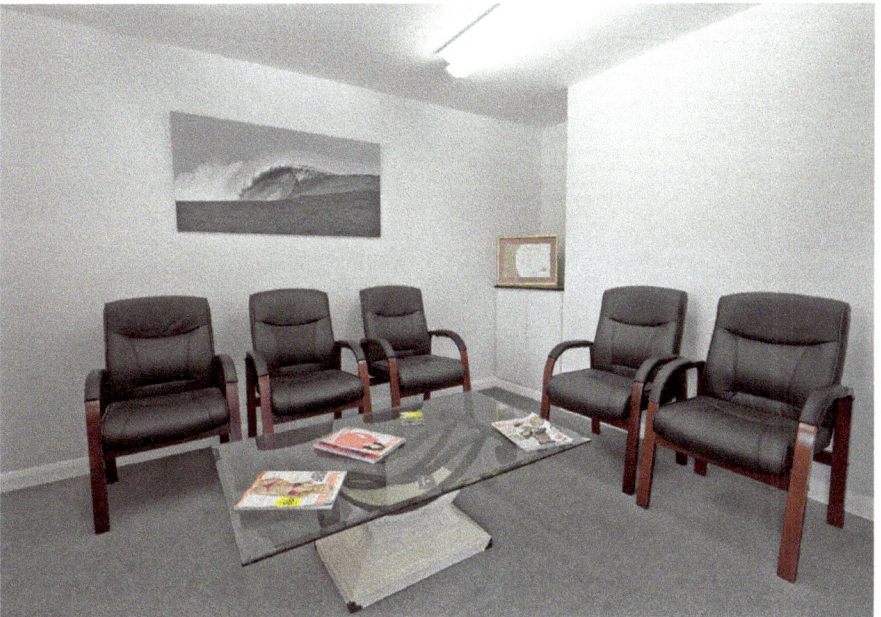

You need a peaceful place wait for your treatment.

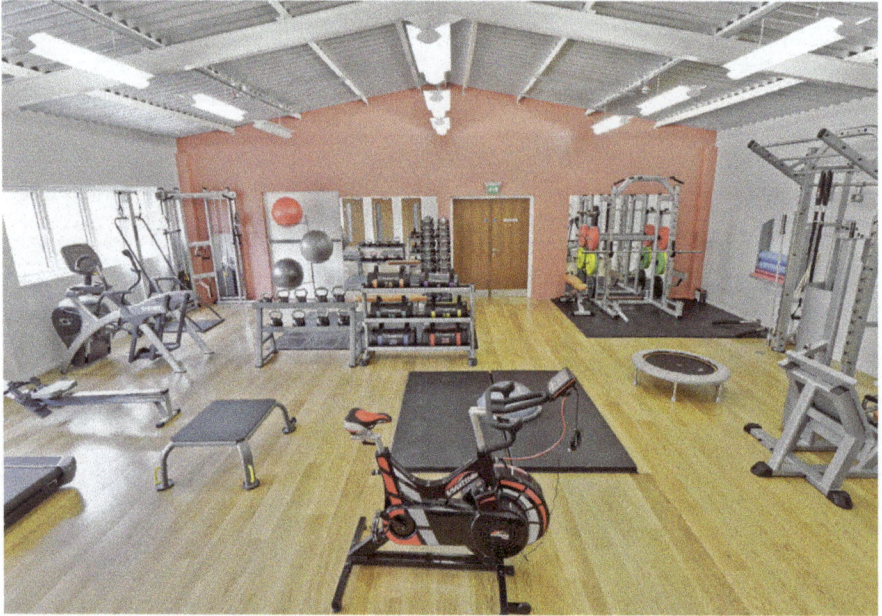

Another view of the gym and rehab space—this is well used by the patients.

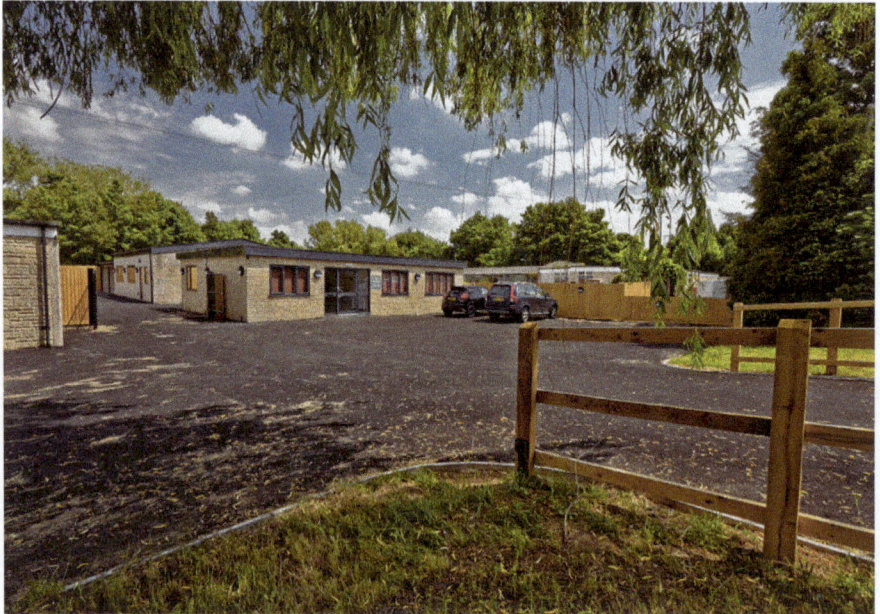

The new beginning finishing and opening the Bosworth Clinic 2013.

6. THE EMERGENT BODY

We see everything from dislocated shoulders to groin, hamstring calf strains to knee and ankle surgeries to low back pain, fractures and spinal surgeries – some of the more common injuries being those to the meniscus, muscles, ligament, tendons, capsules and fascia. Sometimes these injuries, depending on severity, can be treated locally and simply, using a combination of different PRICE processes: protecting, resting, icing, compressing, and elevating.

We may need to offload the area so crutches may be required or an air cast ankle brace. After 48 hours it becomes clearer as to the extent of the injury and then the next steps can be taken to assist the healing and start the process of loading, then players will usually follow a return-to-play plan, and physios will work alongside them to help execute the plan, which may include applying manual-therapy techniques and introducing progressively more difficult exercises using the player's body weight, the strength of their hands and weights. Soon enough, the hope, of course, is that they'll be back outside completing their ball work and fitness drills.

In short, we treat these patients as we would anyone else – but the root is to examine the cause. Why did the ankle turn like that? How can we prevent a future sprain or dislocation? Does the player have any issues and problems that might cause them to become more susceptible to the injury in question? Again, I come back to the idea of detective work. Sometimes injuries occur for no real reason besides normal wear and tear, a bad slip or a fall. However, there's more to be discovered, more to be explored – especially if it's something the player has experienced before.

Rugby is one of the more 'well-known' sports requiring MSK therapy, if I can put it like that! I've worked with the Cornish Pirates team, and London Irish and consulted for few clubs, and both roles have enabled me to understand more of a sport that so often results in fairly serious injury. Rugby combines the fitness and agility needed for football with contact, tackling, force and strength. It is expected that overuse injuries – such as tendonitis, muscle strains and joint sprains, for example – would present often. But there is as much scope for these as for brain injury, however temporary: concussions are common, and the scrumming and rucking required can give rise to all sorts of both acute and chronic problems.

Rugby is at its heart a sport of collision, of impact. And so it stands to reason that we get our fair share of fractures, dislocations and sprains. More common still are bruises, which can sound simple enough until you see how deep into the tissue they can penetrate. Here in the UK, we don't use body pads or helmets either, so there's a decent amount of facial fracturing – jaws, cheekbones and noses, for instance.

Like footballers, rugby players need to be able to change direction quickly – this can result in meniscus tears, in rotational forces placing extreme pressure on ligaments. The shoulders take a real battering in the game, too – imagine two men with a combined weight of 240kg crashing into one another or the ground. We might see a sprain of the acromioclavicular joint (AC separation) or a dislocation of the ball-and-socket glenohumeral joint, one of three/four joints in the shoulder complex.

We can treat the physical injuries well enough, of course, but involvement in a high-pressure, high-intensity job also requires an element of mental diagnosis. The symptoms of concussion might not present for several hours after an injury has occurred, and while we're examining a torn ligament, we might also notice a player's sudden confusion, dizziness, headache or blurred vision. They might appear confused, tetchy or irritable. It is crucial to try and spot the difference between a player who's understandably agitated that they've sustained an injury to one who's in the early stages of a brain injury. Players are now tested on a regular basis for the early signs of concussion these tests are carried out regularly especially if there has been a collision noted by the referee or the medical teams in the stands who are watching specifically for any untoward signs following collisions.

Rugby and football are both fast-moving sports, but it is the former that presents the most opportunity for an injury no one spots. The scrums and rucks provide the perfect screen, in a way, from spectators and referees, and sometimes the chaos of a collision can mask the impact of one player on another or the force with which one hits the ground. It is the physio's job to assess the whole condition, not just the injury that is being presented.

It is difficult, sometimes, to find yourself rubbing up against coaches or players. When you're in charge of teams like this, energy and time can be wasted on politics. It is an immense responsibility, and this is something to bear in mind. One cannot afford to have disruption. It is especially important for younger physios to stand their ground, to speak out if they have concerns and never to be intimidated by the prestige of a team, coach or manager. It's worth remembering that one's training is one's greatest armour in these situations. Naturally, coaches want what is best for their team, but that may come with increased pressure on both them and the players.

'You're all right, aren't you?' they ask fretfully at the side of a patient's bed. It is in no one's interest to keep a player from the field unnecessarily, but it is still more useless to send them back before they're ready.

Another consideration is ability. If, as a physio, you spot a player presenting with the same injuries time after time, the same issues and problems, then it could also be that they are in the wrong place. Is their technique up to scratch? Are they being properly directed and trained? And – most difficult of all to explain – are they in the right team for their ability?

In Canada, some members of our speed skating team were upset with me when I performed the duties I was there, as the physiotherapist, to perform. I informed the squad managers that I would make this easy for them. If I wasn't supported, I'd leave. These experiences can leave you raw, particularly when the weight of expectation sits on your shoulders. In addition, you're often out there alone, abroad, your family back home, working round the clock – and what's more, you're on a massive learning curve.

I was learning every day. But if things went wrong, I was accountable and needed to take the final decision. This, for the physio, can be an immense challenge. At heart, you need to remember you're dealing with someone else's body, with the hopes and dreams – and ego, often – of another person. It's an immense mix of emotion and pressure, but physios need to be prepared to withstand this.

So where do we start? With an insidious onset problem we have no obvious causal link; we are designed to move, therefore, we have to deal with a number of different forces acting on the body but the main two are vertical-ground reaction force and gravity. The first thing to do is to make sure the body is able to accommodate these forces if not correct the reasons for non-compliance and then go look for the problem!

However, in order to go look for the problem you need to understand how the body functions in a 'normal' state and then in a state of specific load, sport or otherwise. Once the block(s) to function has been dealt with the MSK system needs to be re-fired and the muscle timings re-loaded.

Appropriate stimulation needs to be applied at the right time to ensure load management occurs without recourse to dysfunction. Intervention and the intent of the intervention are critical for optimal outcomes. The duration and the intensity of treatment follows a not dissimilar pattern to a coaching program and should be periodised, progressive and structured. Patients must take ownership of their treatment, must be involved in decision making and must be accountable for their decisions. The therapist is the facilitator, advisor and at times will need to take control but always with consent.

Mel Stiff said, "The body has a homeostatic base and is FAR more intelligent than anything we can devise; it will largely reintroduce proper muscle timing if the obstacles are removed. The key is finding the obstacles and using your preferred method to facilitate change and then it's time to get out of the way. Of course, there are variables, and each person is different, but the general paradigm stays the same."

Let's talk about loading. What is load and loading? The Oxford Dictionary defines the term as the 'The application of a mechanical load or force to something' / 'A weight being carried or about to be carried'. How the tissues load and how the body manages these forces is beyond the scope of this first book but it is something that will be discussed at length in the next book.

How is the load managed through the body? Bones, joints, ligaments, muscles, tendons all interdigitating with and as a part of the fascia. What is fascia? 'A thin sheath of fibrous tissue around a muscle or organ'.

The orientation of tissue in the body is continuous. This is important to understand and can be easily seen through dissection. If you can orientate your paradigm towards this thought process, you will more easily monitor changes occurring in one part of the body directly and indirectly affecting other parts. We know the fascia is continuous and can be said to start at bregma on top of the skull ending at the soles of the feet. Much has been written about fascia, many twists and turns, believers and non-believers, but it offers answers. We are only just beginning to know human movement and its many pseudonyms.

Collagen-based time constants are still being investigated but the two we are aware of are sleeping, the body moves everywhere 20 minutes and when standing every third of a second, it's not surprising overload is a problem for when this system starts to fail, not necessarily because of a problem, the whole load management system is affected: a stiff first ray will affect hip joint movement, conversely a loss of fascial mobility at the hip with affect the knee and ankle, but at this stage it's not necessarily a problem, it's just adapting to the change in the 'impulse' (Gracovetsky).

Another important question, where is movement being initiated, what is the quality of the movement and how well is it being controlled. Quality can be defined as the coordinated acceleration and deceleration about the joints requiring a number of actions and tissues to make this happen. Range of movement is not always a good marker of function, although range is specific to the environment in which the body is trying to operate, range without control is not ideal. Remember we train movement not muscle, function is always the priority.

The sacroiliac joint has been an area of contention for years: first they did move and then they didn't move and now they move again but not very much. The important thing to understand is that they do move and how much is different in each individual, accepting there is movement is a fundamental step forward if we are to understand and work with function and performance. Richard Don Tigny has spent a lifetime working with the biomechanics of the sacroiliac joint and the low back, as far back as 1965 he had worked out how the SIJ loaded and affecting function at the low back and hips, he did this through default, as have so many clinicians during that time. There are many other notables who have furthered the cause of sacroiliac joints and pelvic function: Andre Vleeming et al and Diane Lee amongst others.

As therapists, we work with the anatomy, through applied anatomy and biomechanics. It is crucial to know your anatomy and how it applies to 'normal' movement and then to specific sport or activity. Understanding how and why structures become loaded and then overloaded cannot happen if your anatomy is weak. Origins and insertions are not clear-cut: all structures are collagen-based and blend into each other. This is vital for the transmission of forces as well as information. This anatomical dance performed by the tissues in perfect harmony, known as tensegrity, is required for efficient movement, although movement does not necessarily need to be efficient to be effective!! These structures, tissues have been called many things, from chains to slings, but ultimately you must understand what's where and how it responds to the internal and external environmental changes.

The body responds to stress, tissue or tensile stress in different ways and it has mechanisms designed to help us through these situations. Understanding how each individual responds to tissue loading and stress is important for determining how to treat them. The order, intensity and duration of treatment are also dependent on a similar understanding. As a general rule treatment should really be based on minimal effective dose (MED).

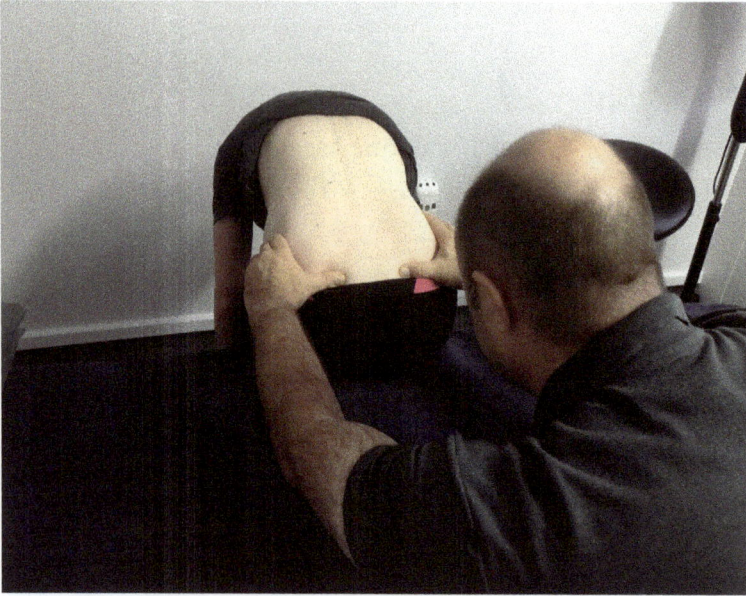

Forward Flexion test, handling skills and visual acuity combined—don't just look at your hands!

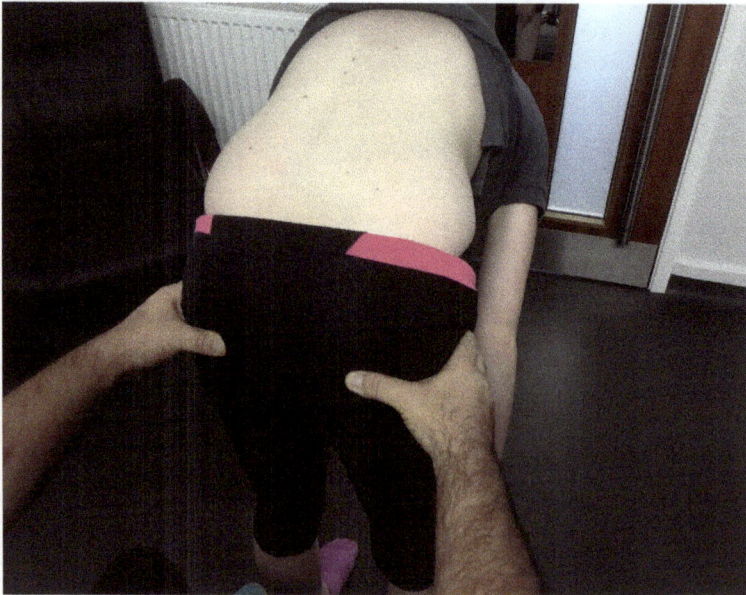

This is an indicator, not overly accurate but you get an idea of relationship between posterior hip and S3 on FF.

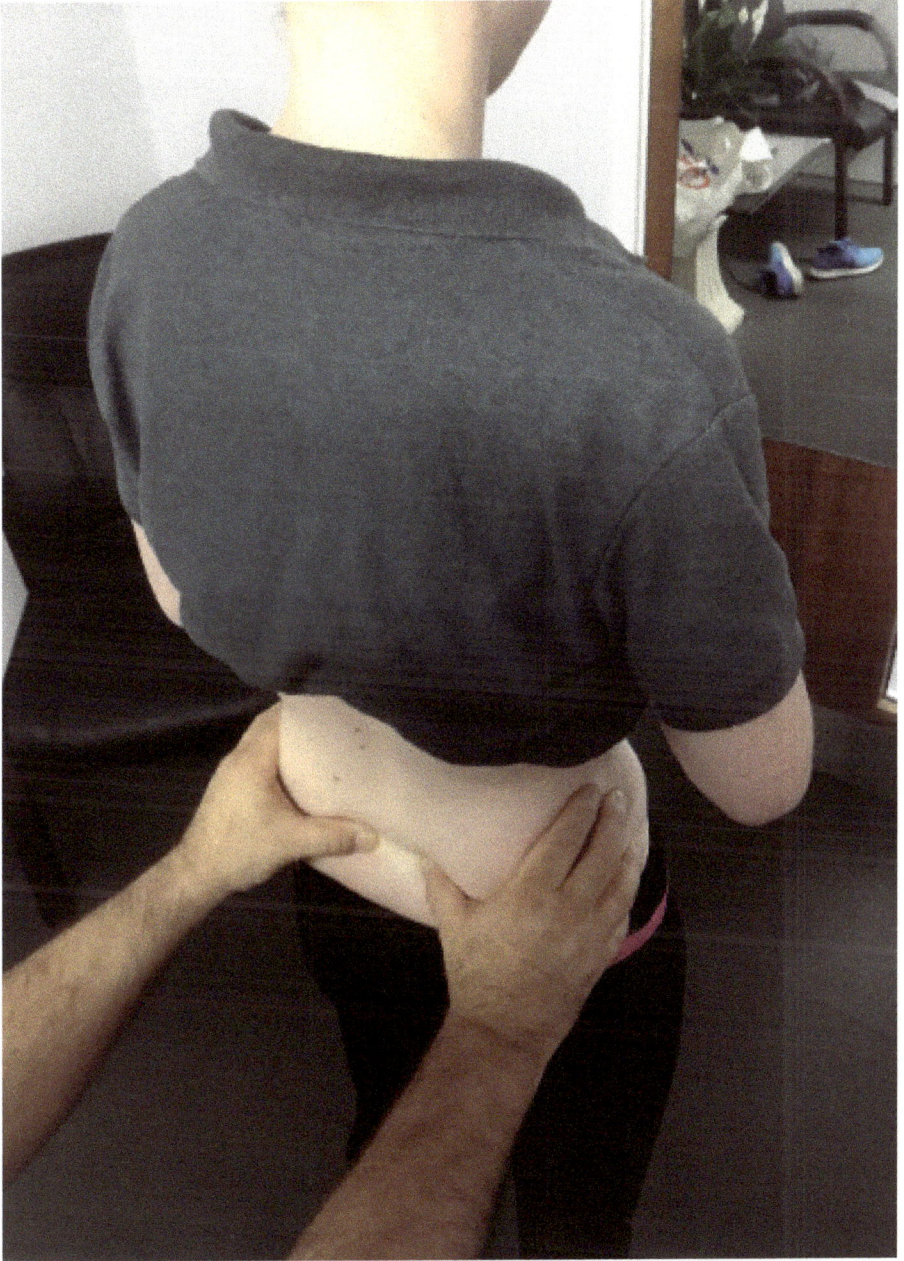

Palpating the sacral sulcii in standing feeling for change on spinal extension.

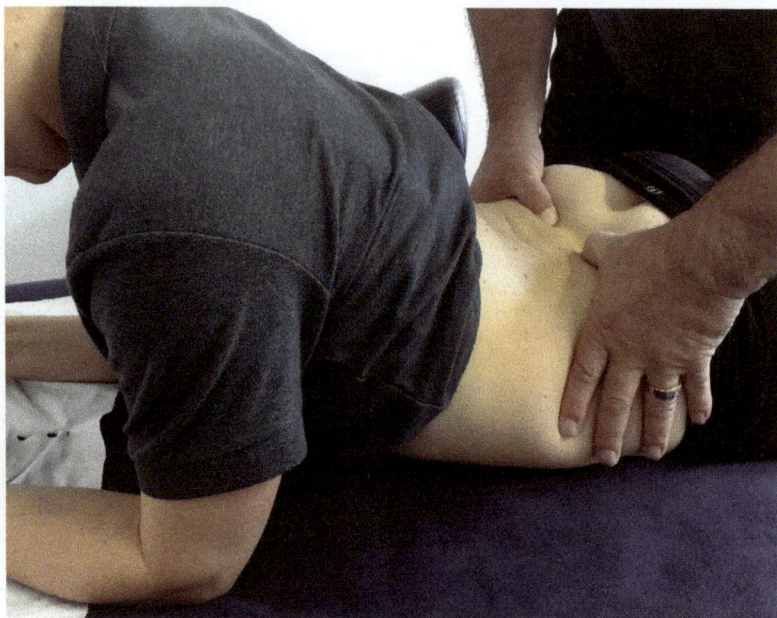

Lumbar spine positional diagnostics when extended.

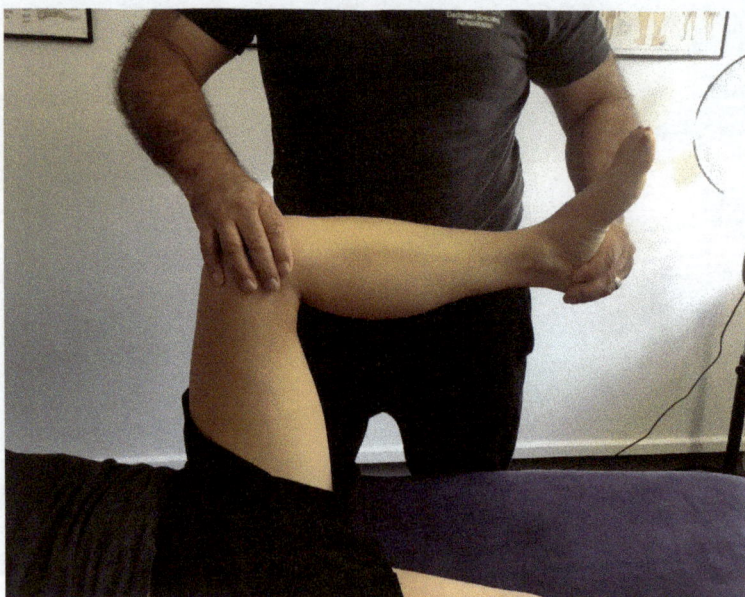

Tibial internal and external rotation, as a general rule, internal should be approx 50% of ext.

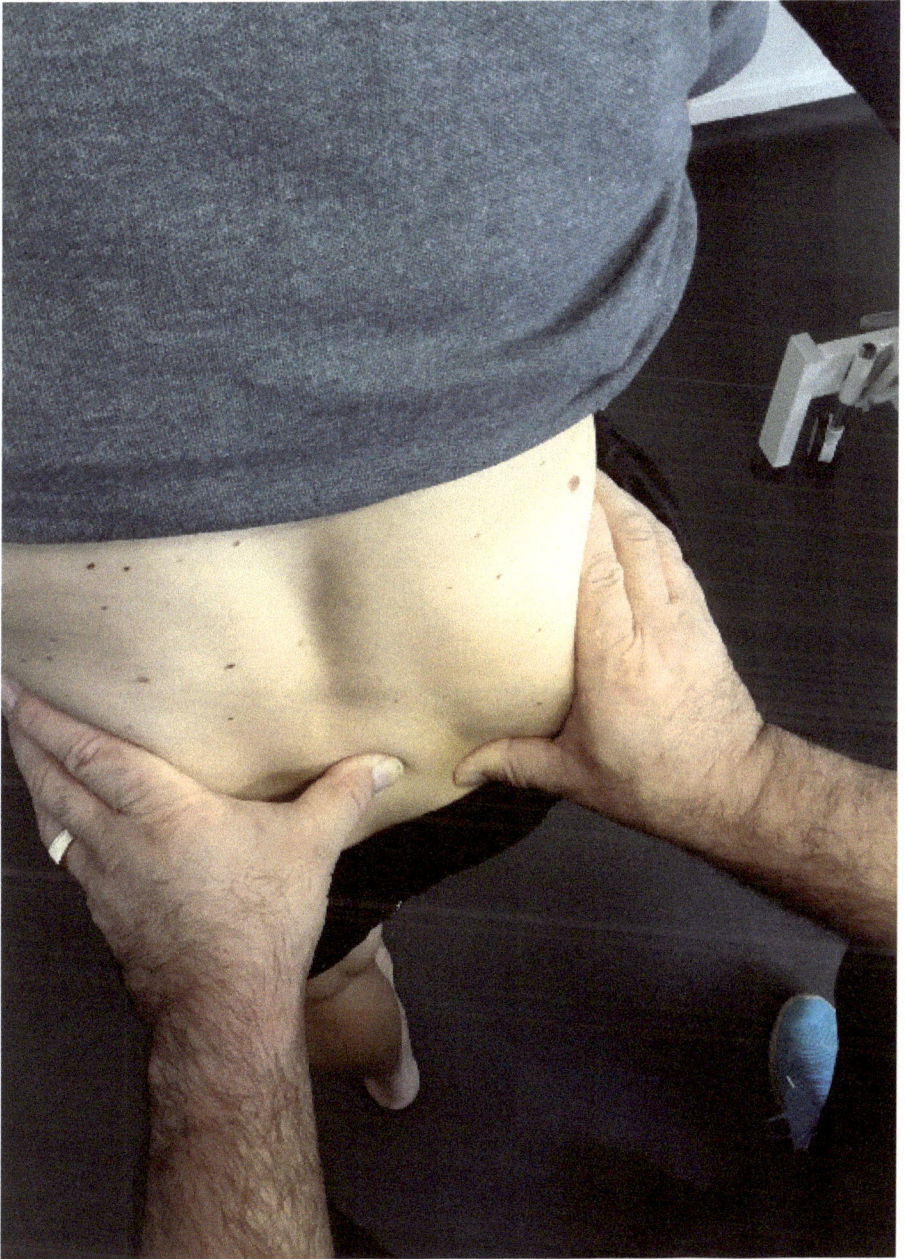

Gillet or Stork test PSIS moves Caudad when functioning 'normally'.

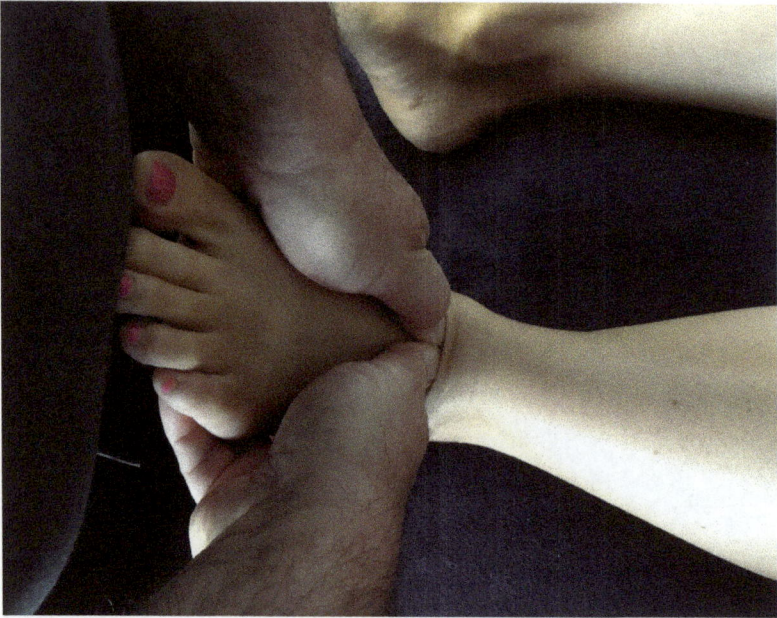

Mobilising the talo-crural joint and making sure it allows dorsi flexion.

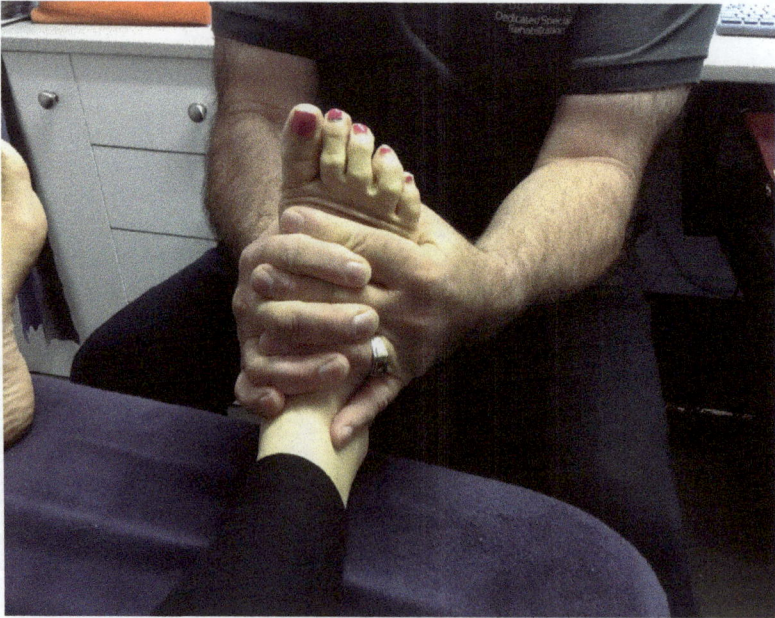

Decompression of the talo-crural joint

7. AN INTEGRATED APPROACH

So how do we take the philosophy outlined earlier and transfer that into examination, reasoning and treatment and how do we measure outcomes? Handling is an essential skill if you are going collect evidence of specific joint/tissue compliance and movement as well as functional movements and responses; I am not referring to movement algorithmic or protocol-driven testing, although we all, in some way, have our way which could be interpreted as a protocol or algorithm?

Many times, our standard tests about the pelvis are not valid because they cannot be evidenced, the truth is the tests are, as a group, valuable in assisting diagnosis but you require a detailed knowledge of your surface anatomy and the ability to locate the landmarks on the body. The reason for these tests not being used by physiotherapist is mainly through a lack of inter-tester reliability resulting from poor handling skills and a movement away from handling being taught as a credible method of working in this modern age of MSK therapy!

Tests like standing spinal forward flexion tests, seated spinal flexion tests, Stork or Gillet test, sacral positional testing do give you a picture as to what is not moving or functioning appropriately for the particular patient. You need to understand through your questioning and knowledge of the mechanism and your patients thoughts what the various 'bandwidths' (McMillan) are about the joints and tissues.

These bandwidths give you a feel for how they should move and how they are moving. Remember, earlier I mentioned if you don't know what is supposed to happen or how a joint, limb body is supposed to move how do you know when it's not moving properly? It's this lack of understanding that often leads to the statement that these tests are 'not valid' – sadly this happens all too often and consequently patients do not improve or their problems are merely moved to another part of their body. Obviously, experience, anecdotal and pragmatic evidence are our allies for the most part but there is some evidence out there to assist. The problem with insidious onset problems is that they are not clear and are generally multi-factorial and complex to set up RCTs should be difficult and costly and there does not appear to be a will to do so. Therapists/healers have been handling bodies for millennia, I could use the following example - when a child falls and hurts themselves we do not give them an exercise that might have been evidenced we rub or stoke the area Just a thought!

Key factors in the accurate use of these tests start with your hands being symmetrical when on the body otherwise you cannot see the movement. As your experience grows you will eventually learn to feel the movement occurring and really start to see what and how the body is initiating the movement. Handing pressure is also important: too much pressure and you will affect the tissue and the test will be invalid – placement of the hands is paramount – this is the single biggest reason for the tests failing to give useful information.

Further information can be gathered whilst the patient is standing: note whether they are standing with their feet under their shoulders and whether the weight is equally transferred through both legs, also where is the weight felt in the feet, central, towards the heels or towards the toes. If the legs are wider than the shoulders this could indicate some loss of form closure (as described by Vleeming et al) at the SIJ, the body needs to increase the force through the hip via the femoral neck into the S3 region which aligns with the acetabulum. Similarly, if the weight is more through one leg than the other, although there may be several reasons for this. If the weight is towards the heels again they are attempting to increase the posterior chain force to increase form closure or SIJ loading capacity.

Again, the body needs to be efficient in order to utilise energy in the most cost-effective way as in standing and easy ambulant gait there is little muscle activation required to control the load, therefore, when there is an increased amount of muscle activation in and around the hips and pelvis this could indicate a loss of efficient form closure. Gravity is a constant so the forces pushing down to the ground don't change however, VGRF does. In order to remain efficient and effective and cope with increasing VGRF, we need to increase muscle actions from the long two joint muscles and the various slings: these will increase stability and function and allow us to transfer greater loads.

The standing flexion test (SFT) give you some idea of how the ilium is moving on the sacrum. Place your hands symmetrically on the posterior superior iliac spines (PSIS) and hook your thumbs on the inferior surface as the patient flexes forward the thumbs should remain at the same level, if there is any form of dysfunction one will look as though it is moving upwards as the sacral attempts to relatively counter nutate. It is possible for both SIJs to be problematic, but one will tend to show more than the other.

Standing Extension test to see if the lumbar spine is rotating left or right on movement which means there is some side-bend and rotation occurring to the same side at one or more of the lumbar segments which stops the smooth flow of the cardinal movement into extension. The same can be said for spinal flexion if the movement is not smooth and flowing it is usually because there is some segmental dysfunction. Clearly, no dysfunction occurs on its own there are always a number of components as nothing in the body works in isolation.

S3 Posterior hip, fingers on the GT and the thumbs placed in the glute approximately at the posterior hip level in line with the GT; when flexing forward do the thumbs stay level or is one thumb moving upwards, this is a test I designed to give me further information on how the body is dealing with the load through the hips when bending forwards and bringing the pelvis into anterior tilt.

Passive Hip Extension Prone, knee flexed hand on area of the glute around posterior hip or at the base of the spine left and right side to restrict spinal extension as much as possible, some is okay as long as you apply same force, direction and control to each side, this is again just an indicator of the tension through the anterior chain.

What sets athletes apart from the general population? It would be more accurate to ask what doesn't. Athletes are a world of difference from your average person, even the fittest among us, the weekend warriors and marathon runners. For most people sport is a hobby, a necessary part of life for sure, but not a job. They don't make money from it or have tight schedules revolving around it, and they don't need expert guidance on extraordinary musculoskeletal issues. They head to the gym when time allows, they lift weights or see a personal trainer, they play a game of five-a-side and hit the showers. For most of us, exercise is a pleasurable and endorphin-releasing pastime.

I work with athletes, by contrast, who are trained to perform very specific functions, trained to use specific skills. They require the most tailored of approaches, the most nuanced training plans. We need to understand their bodies in the context of the exercise they're doing. And while many athletes will specialise in a particular area, a swimmer (for example) might still complete running practice, cross-training or gym-based practice in any given week. Their stress points will be totally different to that of our average client.

I might see a skater, for instance, with stress points on the front of their hip or on their abductors – they're bent over double going round the track at 60kph, for instance. For sprinters, their stress points will change depending on how they're hitting the ground. Their feet, tibia, upper leg, thighs and glutes. These are the areas that take on the most damage, the most force and pressure. If the system on top of the feet is working optimally, then the stress is much easier to cope with. If it isn't optimised, then that stress causes problems in the lower limb. For boxers there will be different areas – their bodies take on stress day by day, in the way they move but also how they're hit and where. They are also dealing with rapid rotational forces which again need to be controlled, otherwise they can be vulnerable to injury.

Understanding these different sports is critical to a holistic examination of a problem for any given athlete. What is also important to note is that in order for the athlete to perform effectively, certain areas will be tighter than others – the body sometimes has to function within an area of tightness, within an environment that's conducive to the athlete's given sport.

We need to be constantly aware of the environments they're working in, too. We might look at the external training environment, suggesting ways in which this might change to accommodate better healing. We might suggest to coaches and trainers that change will enhance performance. If an athlete isn't full-time, we might suggest that their working environment – sitting hunched over a computer for hours at a time – might need to be altered to change the ergonomics of the body. We see more and more people using standing desks, which make a huge difference to the lower back and the neck. It's all about optimisation, at the end of the day.

Another important factor for consideration is the differences between types of treatment when it comes to athletes. We may watch a tennis or football match and see the medics running onto the court or pitch, the First Aid bag held aloft. These acute injuries need immediate attention: the cuts and scrapes, the falls. But physios working on the night following an Olympic event or on the morning of that event are looking to optimise an athlete's performance for that specific day and time. It's a very different approach to the longer-term, more holistic therapy we might be advocating for with patients in our clinics.

If an athlete runs into difficulties during a sporting event but is well enough to continue participating, they need their particular problem addressed in the moment. They need their body to be assessed and adjusted to help give the performance they expect to deliver. Once the games are finished, we can focus on more broad-brush rehabilitation – most athletes will give it their all during their heat or race and will require intervention afterwards. And this makes our job all the more difficult, since we're treating the problem in the short term and turning to the rehab much later, once the athletes returned home and gone back to their usual training programme.

Sometimes, too, it's important to realise there can be resistance to an outside physio. The pressure can be enormous, and teams might go outside their comfort zone for new blood. If medals aren't being won, something might be wrong.

Case in point: at the Vancouver games, the culture was different to what I had anticipated. The Canadians are non-confrontational by nature, and therefore to avoid any issues I found they sometimes didn't tell me everything I needed to know. My use of language, too, and the ease with which I addressed people, it felt out of place. There was a more straight-talking system in the UK, and it took me a bit of time to adjust to this new landscape.

In UK athletics, the process was different. I was back in the UK after the games and was offered the role of chief physio for the UK's track team, a huge honour. Here's a lesson. You may feel underprepared, and you may feel each day that you're climbing the Eiger – but do it. If you've been approached for a specific job that you want but don't feel up to, it's important to take it if you can. The experience will add years to your professional expertise.

I was learning again now – this time about track. I spent hours in the evenings with coaches, learning an enormous amount each and every night. I needed to find a way to bring everyone together through a variety of strategies. Track and field can very much get under the skin. It's one of the toughest and most exacting, sports I have worked in because you must be precise. And as a result, I became a better therapist for having been involved with this area.

I am most proud of the fact that when I took over, we had a high percentage of injured athletes in London and Loughborough. I brought this down massively, not through incredible clinical treatment but by altering the culture in the medical team and the way they communicated with the coaching staff. Medical staff often, I found, could appear to talk down to coaches. It was entirely non-conducive as a paradigm. This approach to communication was important to me, and once the coaches began to realise these were conversations, not directives, injury rates came down. That was a healthy shift – talking, teamwork, rather than magical clinical skills really started to make a difference. I didn't want to suggest how people performed MSK therapy, but I did want to encourage talking *with* someone rather than *at* them. The way we communicate in multi-disciplinary teams is really important.

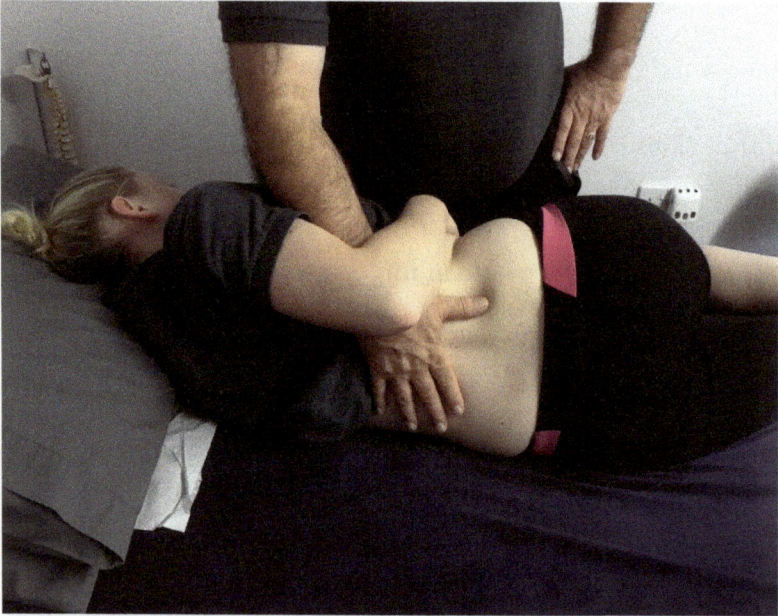

Setting up to adjust the lower lumbar spine.

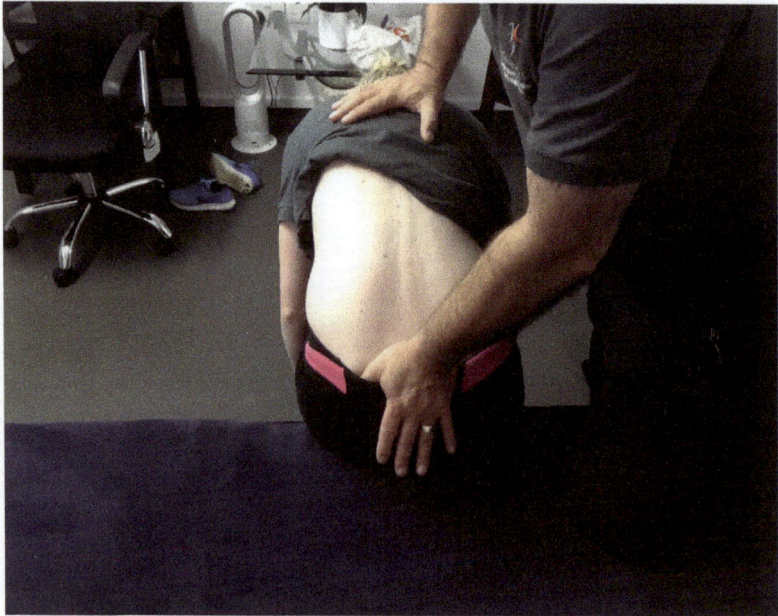

Myotactic activation procedure for a bilateral flexed sacrum.

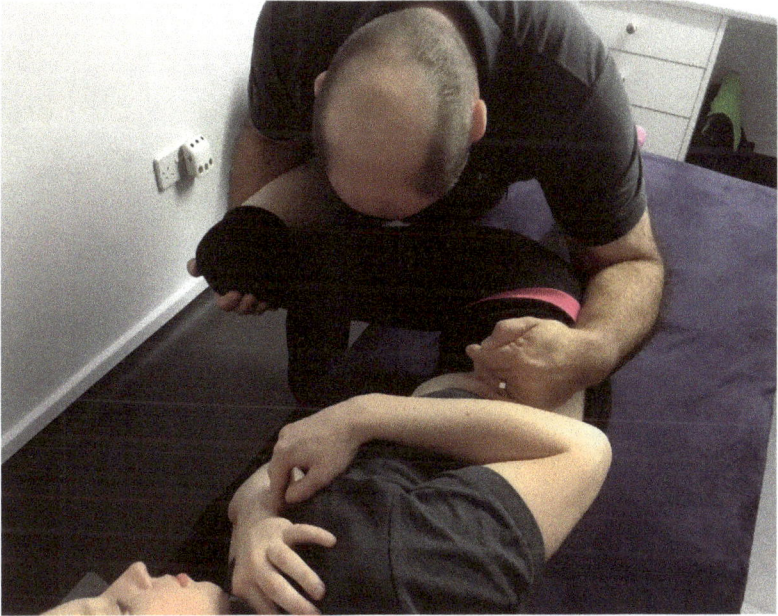

Myotactic activation procedure for an anterior rotated ilium.

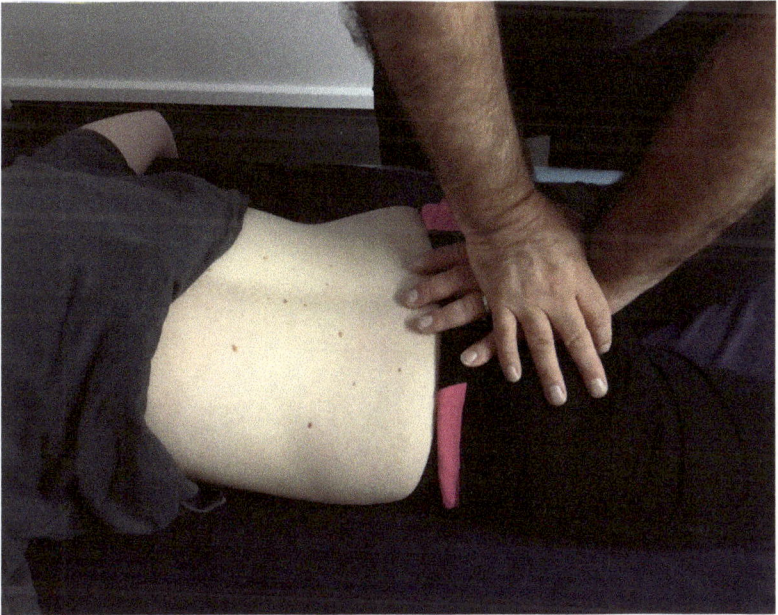

Sacral spring and myotactic activation procedure for Unilateral sacral flexion.

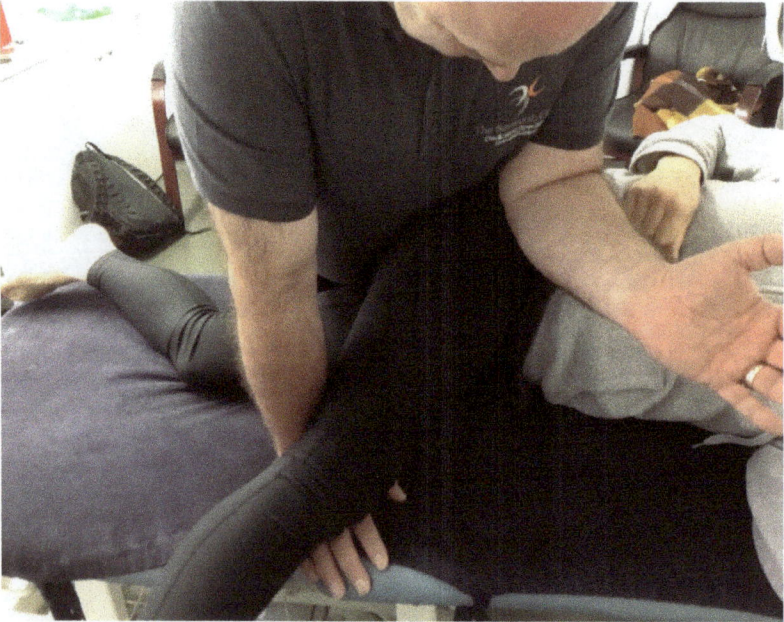

Active Release TFL.

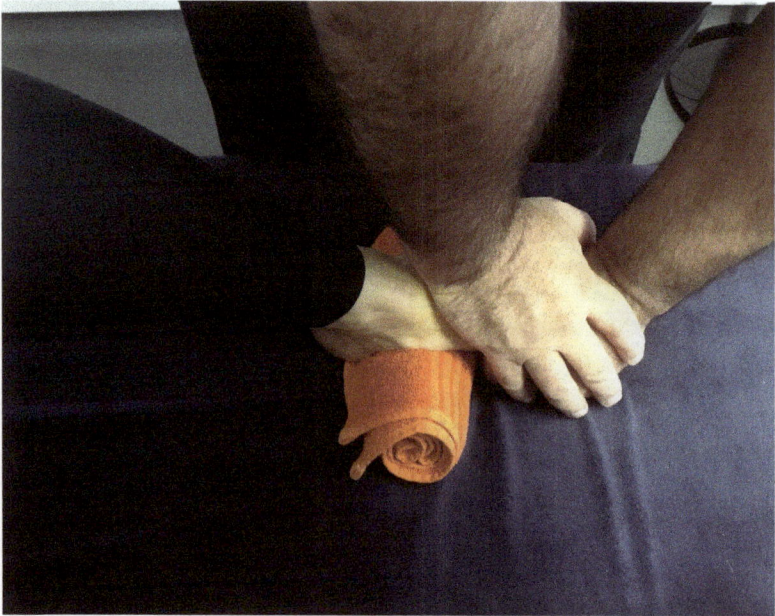

Mobilisation of the first ray.

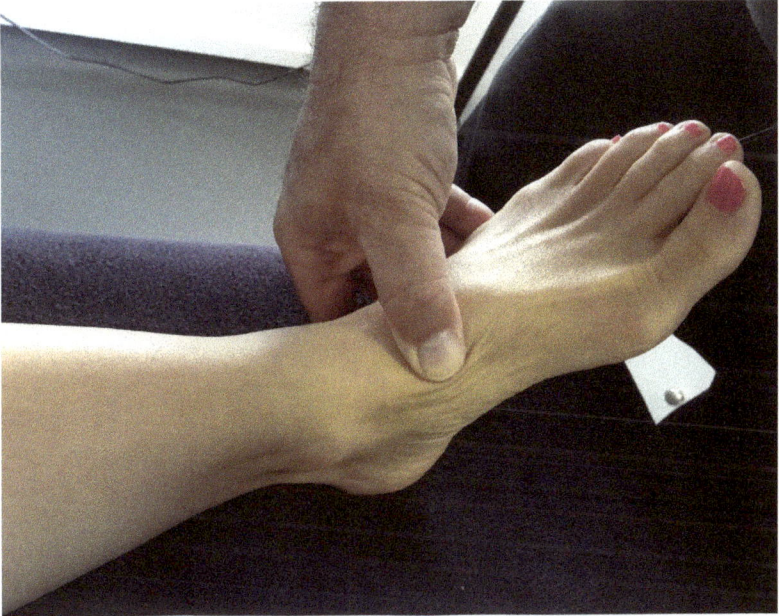

Navicular important bone and prone to stress reactions and fractures.

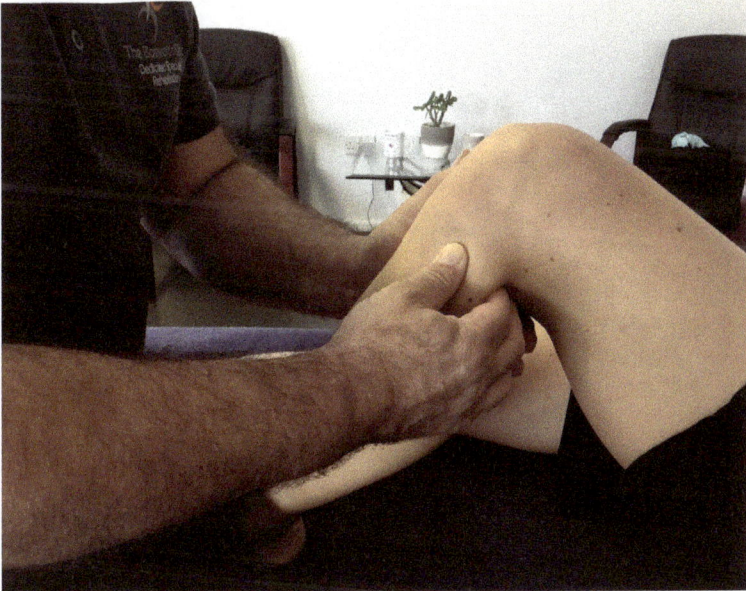

Very important joint the Superior Tib Fib Joint. Affects tibial and hip rotation as well as loading through the limb.

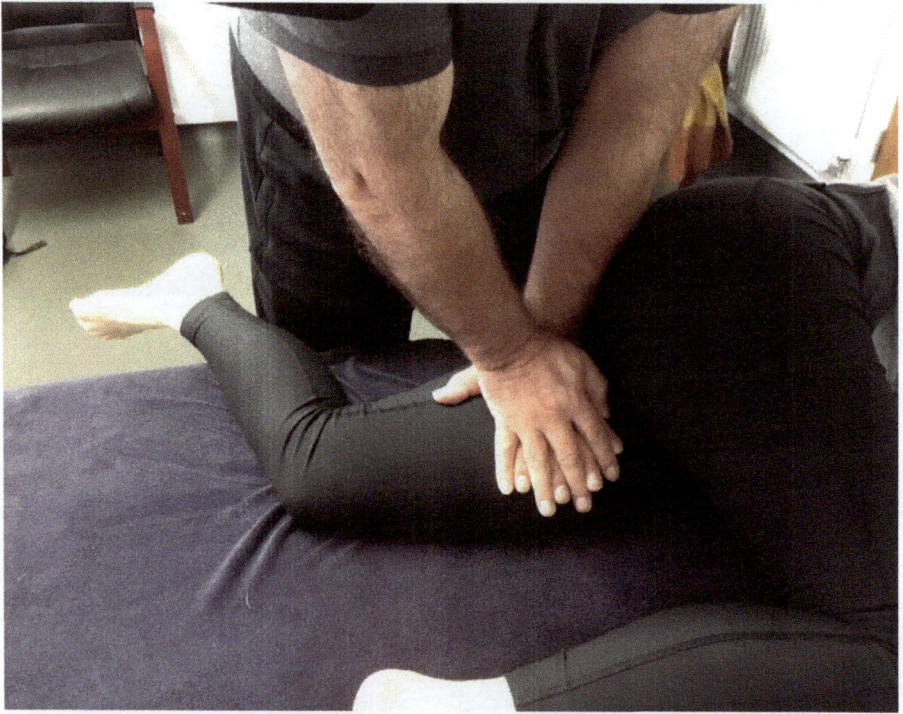

Deep tissue release at the Adductor compartment.

8. THE NEXT GENERATION

Physiotherapists entering the profession nowadays will receive many hundreds of hours of training. They will need to complete a degree-level qualification in MSK therapy either as an undergraduate or as a two-year Master's degree. Once this is completed, the trainee must register with the Health and Care Professions Council, or HCPC.

Modern-day MSK therapy training places a strong emphasis on developing high-quality analytical skills to assess the robustness and applicability of research in order to effectively integrate it into practice. In addition, foundational knowledge of strength and conditioning is provided, with a focus on utilising guidelines established by the American College of Sports Medicine (ACSM). However, it is important to note that hands-on skills in MSK therapy training are primarily limited to assessment techniques rather than treatment techniques. This shift is driven by the growing emphasis on evidence-based practice, where manual therapy techniques and modalities with limited research backing are discouraged. It should be clarified that physiotherapists are not taught to be completely hands-off, but in a National Health Service (NHS) setting, where time is limited and efficiency is key, exercise therapy has been proven beneficial through research and is therefore prioritised as a primary treatment approach.

Why might a young person, or indeed a not-so-young one, decide to become a physio, and what sorts of qualities do they need to have? Most importantly, physios are healers. They would have no work without people, so they need to be empathetic, kind, open-minded and non-judgemental. You might, in the course of an average day, have appointments with a 20-year-old professional footballer, an 80-year-old ex-nurse, a child with walking difficulties, a young man with a grade-three sprained ankle, a young woman with a recently reconstructed knee. It's a job that requires an enormous amount of patience, problem-solving capabilities and a reassuring and practical approach.

Most crucially, physios need to be good listeners, care about the conditions of their patients and be willing to accept that not all programmes of treatment will necessarily result in a 'solving' of the problem. To this end, they need to be excellent communicators, as happy listening to a colleague's opinion as voicing their own. They'll need to be able to explain things to patients, to really try and discuss in layman's terms why a particular course of action might help or might not. We don't have the answers, though, we merely facilitate.

And when things don't go the way anyone intended, they need to be able to try another course – to motivate the patient and go again. It seems an obvious point, but physios really need to be physically fit as well – the work can be intense and demanding.

On the academic side, physiotherapists will usually require two or three A levels, including one in biological science and/or one in PE. This will be in addition to five GCSEs between grades A and C. Nonetheless, there are other routes, such as BTECs, HNDs or HNCs, relevant NVQs or a full practising qualification in a related area. One of the best pieces of advice for someone considering entering the field is to spend some time working with a physio: actually go out and experience the day-to-day, the one on one, and see if you like it. After you've finished your studies, you'll be able to register as a practitioner. This is where you'll also submit an annual retention fee and promise to keep your knowledge and skills up to date.

If I'm honest, I think many physios graduating today would do well to learn in a more hands-on, practical environment. It is all very well taking on the best and brightest new minds to enter the profession, but they will be little use without direct experience. It takes a lifetime to become a really good physio or sports physio, and those years of work gradually build confidence and spell success. Young physios just out of university may be incredibly intelligent, and I don't doubt that they are, but that intelligence is nothing if they're not able to apply their skills with their hands. I had a great deal of hands-on time as a trainee, and I feel that nowadays the young receive next to nothing by comparison. You need the skills to back up the training.

Let's take the example of a hamstring tear. We need evidence to show how a particular exercise programme might or might not help. Of course we do. But we also need to understand why the hamstring problem happened in the first place: that's the key question. We won't necessarily optimize the outcome if we work only on a completely evidence-based model. Unfortunately, evidence-based practice generally follows the flowchart of possibilities to the letter, and sometimes patients would benefit from a different approach. It's important to state, too, that physios should use an evidence-based, pragmatic and anecdotal combination as the best of all approaches.

Let's not forget that the history of MSK therapy revolves around moving patients with hands, with massage, with handling the body. If you don't touch your patient, you won't do any harm, but you won't do any good either.

I am entirely sympathetic to the issues newly qualified physiotherapists face and will continue to face. The recent Covid pandemic have made our work significantly more difficult. Many routine operations were cancelled as a result of the pandemic, delaying post-operative recovery and rehabilitation and often exacerbating existing medical or musculoskeletal problems. We were barely able to practise at all during the worst days: our jobs require face-to-face interaction and a hands-on approach, both of which were advised against during the strictest phases of lockdown.

Of course, we could conduct Zoom consultations, but the limitations of technology have made that a challenge. We need to be able to see our patients' movement – or lack thereof – without the interruptions of WiFi issues and glitches.

If it was hard for myself and my team, it must have been doubly difficult for trainees. The first days of any new job are intimidating, but they must have been much more so for those tasked with making people well again. It is a hugely responsible position to find oneself in. For hospital physios, too, seeing patients intubated and ventilated and spending days locked inside personal-protective equipment must have been incredibly tough. Suddenly you're on-call and anything might happen. Physios in casualty would have seen all manner of deeply unwell patients arrive and sometimes, tragically, never leave.

In addition, physios and therapy-support workers are in short supply at present. The problem we face now is the post-Brexit world of work visas and a points-based system that will not guarantee entry for new clinicians in the NHS. At the same time, post-Covid rehab needs are soaring. We know that the virus has affected every age group and demographic and that the effects of long Covid can be felt for many months if not years after infection.

The Bosworth Clinic, my own workplace, is a teaching clinic, and we regularly hold CPD training, as well as one-to-one mentoring and courses. This is quite common among private clinics. Nowadays, I also serve as a mentor to several medical teams, including ALTIS and UKA, as well as various medical and S&C professionals. I think all physios have to walk the walk, not just talk the talk. We have to pave the way for the next generation, trying to inspire them, opening up our clinics and offices to welcome them indoors for a look.

I strongly believe, too, that if a particular clinic or group of clinics is doing good work, it's incumbent on them to share it. I believe that, due to years of experience, my team has excellent insights on areas that some physios don't work with, especially those in the NHS. Our focus on insidious-onset-type issues and performance-related issues, I think, fits us into a smaller group of physios.

There's nothing so important as inspiring the next generation. Somewhere, somehow, every single physiotherapist – myself included – was inspired to enter the profession. This might have been as a result of childhood issues or illness, as was the case with Dr Janda, or after speaking to a teacher, family friend or similar about the industry. Young people nowadays know that so many jobs will, over the next century or so, become more and more prone to automation. I think that MSK therapy – which will always be performed by humans, as so much of it requires intuition above all else – is one of the safest career paths open to them.

And what's more, it's the best job in the world.

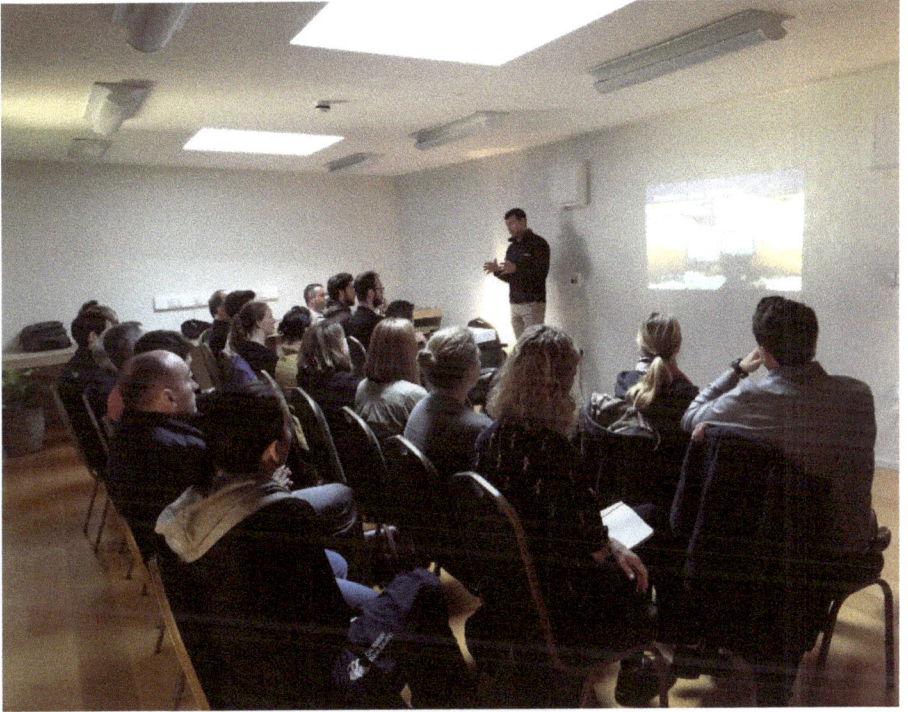

My team educating the up and coming and slightly longer in the tooth Therapists on all things Triathlon.

CONCLUSIONS

For the past 40 years, I've been fortunate enough to do a job that I love. I've worked with the highest-ranking sporting professionals in the country, with sports teams watched by millions around the world and with members of the general, non-sporting public who simply want to improve the quality of their lives. It's ever varied, ever interesting. It's kept me and my team occupied, anyway! I mentioned that MSK therapy is a lot like detective work. We can also think about it as a mass of tangled wires. Everyone has that drawer in their house filled with random cables, charging points, wires: we keep them, and over time they become scrambled, impossible to see clearly. It's our job to pull out these threads, slowly and carefully, from the ground up. It's like rebuilding: we need to assess what the damage is to the best of our ability, and then – only then – do we put plans in place to gently correct it.

The body is designed to move. It copes with load each and every day, with the force of gravity and with contact or surface forces. Gravity is a constant, as we know. It pushes down every moment of our waking and sleeping lives. But the vertical ground reaction force is its diametric opposite. Whether we're walking, running, jumping or climbing – all of these activities change the load and determine whether we'll be in trouble or not.

The body is designed to be incredibly efficient: it hates inefficiency. However, it doesn't necessarily need to be efficient to be effective. Tissue doesn't like to be overloaded, and when it is, it changes its characteristics. Soon enough the body, in turn, begins to change its habits, adapting to its new normal – even if this isn't conducive to optimum muscle use. After a certain amount of time, though, it'll start to send out pain signals. So if we can remove the 'why?' – the idea of overload – then the pain will go, because there's literally no requirement for it.

We need to manage load and understand where it's coming from, the target tissue and performance angle. I might meet a boxer, for instance, and that interaction, that assessment, will by default need to take in everything I understand about the load of a boxer when he or she moves. I'll need to focus on key areas of his system and assess how he can optimise them. Here's the thing: with the body, we can get away with murder in our 20s and a reasonable amount in our 30s. By the time we hit our 40s, however, things get trickier. The body begins to degenerate – albeit slowly – from around the age of 25. We are considered optimum at the age of 25.

We all have our memories of being able to run, jump, hop and skip with abandon as a child, the way we'd tear round playgrounds or sports fields without ceasing for hours on end. Lethargy hits in adolescence as hormones go into overdrive, but by the time we reach 17 or 18, we're in our prime again. For around the next decade, we are ready for anything the world throws at us. The statistical likelihood of causing damage to oneself during this time is also proportionally higher of course. We take greater risks, we feel invincible, we imagine ourselves to be Superman or Superwoman.

It's for this reason that I'd advise younger people to invest in their musculoskeletal health early. Even for just a few weeks, a strength and conditioning coach can work wonders. They'll assess you, identify areas of weakness and explain how to keep your body in the best possible shape. It can be enormously useful in preventing long-standing problems from developing later down the line.

And it's becoming ever more important. For the vast majority of us, our working lives are sedentary. We're sat down for hours and hours on end, staring at a screen. And after a week of minimal movement, we expect our bodies to thank us when we rise on a Saturday and lift weights for two hours or run 13 miles without breakfast. We need to realise that the body is designed to move and that it needs to move often. Any exercise is better than none, of course, but it's no use, really, doing nothing for a week and then throwing everything at one overlong run. You're much more likely to injure yourself this way.

The majority of our clients are over the age of 50, and the demographic tends to be those from a higher-earning socioeconomic background. I am committed to helping whoever books into our clinic while also reflecting on the uncomfortable fact that it shouldn't take a decent insurance package or very deep pockets to be able to afford the best sort of care.

We have a fairly even split of male and female patients, which is heartening, and which means the team can continue to expand their knowledge. Sometimes certain systems and issues are sex-specific, so it helps to see this wide range of the population. I must confess I'm often astonished at women's internal pain tolerance – though of course sometimes this can be a hindrance. I may have to ask a female patient several times to confirm the severity of her pain, and it's only much later in our discussions that she discloses just how bad it's been.

I am grateful to have had a lifetime's career in this industry, learning every day, trying to decipher the many codes and symbols the body presents in all its forms. Ultimately I want to ensure my patients take the route to a better life, to show them that – despite often decades of pain – they needn't continue to put up with what they've experienced before. The cycle can change if we look at the body cohesively and try our best. When I begin my interventions, I have to point out that sometimes I won't know why something is happening, and if that's the case, I won't touch it. But I will do my best to find out. There is nothing so endlessly fascinating as the human body, so consistently surprising. Again, I come back to that idea of detective work, of finding the fault, of looking to the first piece of evidence, the direct cause and effect.

I'm 64 now, and receiving emails – 'I can't wait to come back in', 'thank you so much', 'I've never seen results like these' – as I occasionally do makes it all worthwhile. It is so incredibly rewarding. When I'd been qualified for 10–12 years, I was working so hard and getting so frustrated. Dr Janda changed everything for me in the mid-'90s, and I was mesmerised. I don't think I'd be where I am today without this knowledge. But I sought it out, in a way: we were on a weekend course, after all. I would advise young physios to seek out these experiences, to try and find their own mentor, their own inspiring figure in the industry. There are turning points like this in all our lives. If you do not understand what *should* happen, you're just being led by symptoms in a world of insidious onset. What an epiphany.

The training all physios receive will encompass the need to do no harm — it is important, vital, even, to ask the body questions and allow it to facilitate the answers. I see treatment as a physical question rather than an answer. We give it exercises to do or manoeuvre it in a certain way, but we remain humble before it — we listen to it. Remember, the patient's body knows far more about what it requires to get better than we do. It holds the answers, so we must find and ask the right questions.

The End

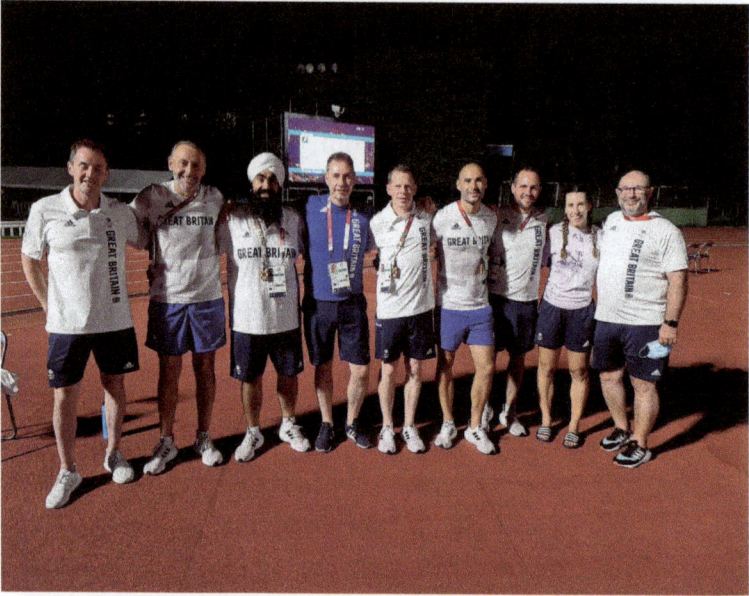

The Medical Team who worked hard at the Tokyo Olympic Games to keep the Athletes competitive.

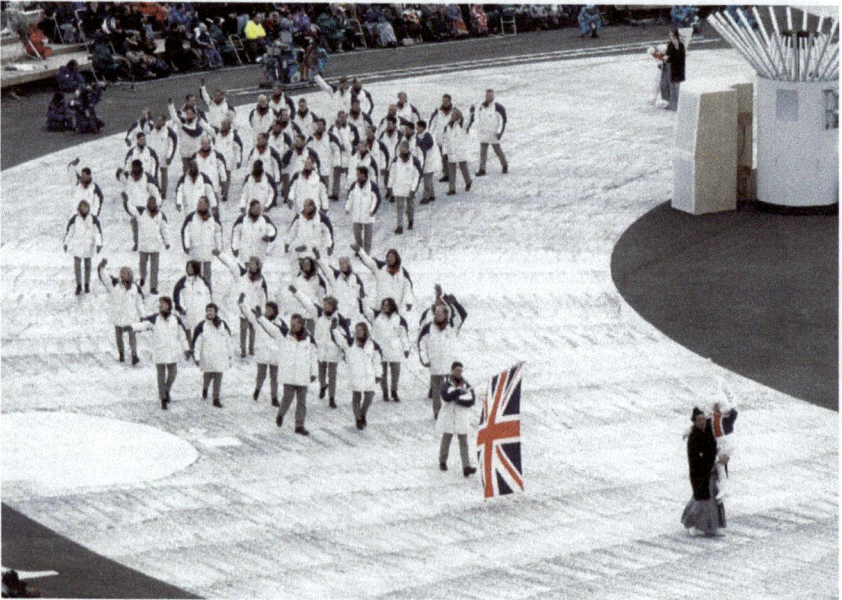

This is where it started 1998 Nagano Olympic Games. I am at the back bringing up the rear.

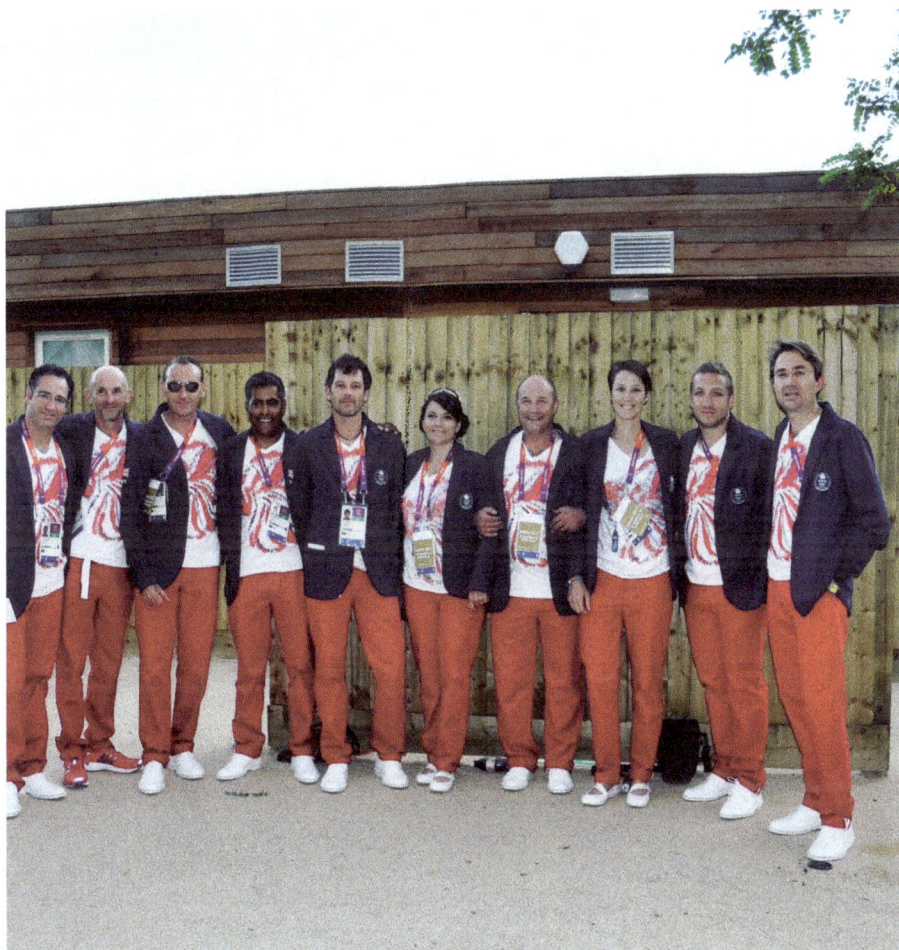

The 2012 London Olympic Games Track and Field Medical team: a very talented group of doctors and therapists.

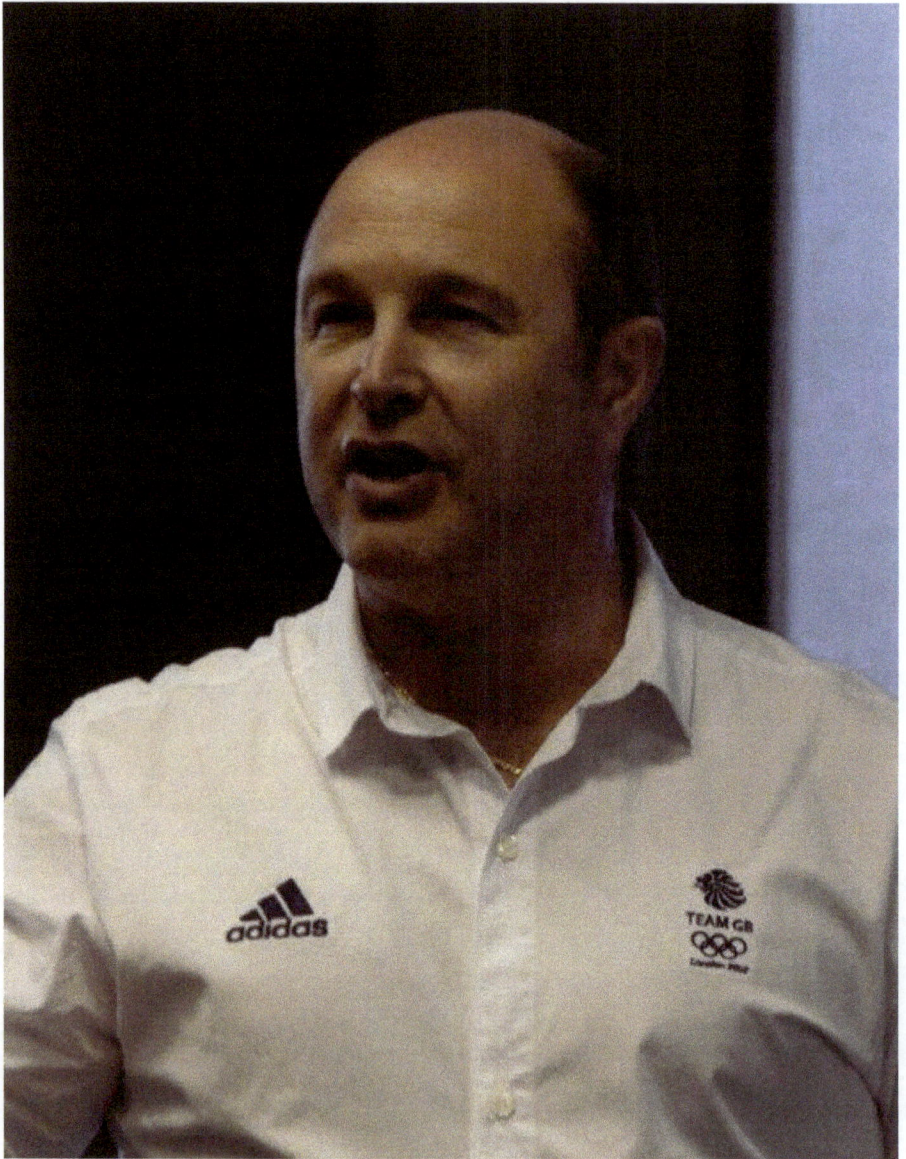

Older but hopefully wiser; remember what we have learned over the last 100 years and use our hands not just our brains.

Milton Keynes UK
Ingram Content Group UK Ltd.
UKHW020753160224
437943UK00002B/24

9 781738 449026